REHABILITATING AMERICA

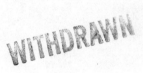

Other books by Frank Bowe

Handicapping America: Barriers to Disabled People

Coalition Building

Planning Effective Advocacy Programs

Rehabilitating America

TOWARD INDEPENDENCE FOR DISABLED AND ELDERLY PEOPLE

FRANK BOWE

HARPER & ROW, PUBLISHERS

NEW YORK

Cambridge
Hagerstown
Philadelphia
San Francisco

1817

London
Mexico City
São Paulo
Sydney

REHABILITATING AMERICA: TOWARD INDEPENDENCE FOR DISABLED AND ELDERLY PEOPLE. Copyright © 1980 by Frank Bowe. All rights reserved. Printed in the United States of America. No part of this book may be used or reproduced in any manner whatsoever without written permission except in the case of brief quotations embodied in critical articles and reviews. For information address Harper & Row, Publishers, Inc., 10 East 53rd Street, New York, N.Y. 10022. Published simultaneously in Canada by Fitzhenry & Whiteside Limited, Toronto.

FIRST EDITION

Designer: Sidney Feinberg

Library of Congress Cataloging in Publication Data

Bowe, Frank.
   Rehabilitating America.
   Bibliography: p.
   Includes index.
   1. Physically handicapped—Rehabilitation—United States. 2. United States—Social policy. I. Title.
HV3023.A3B68   1980   362.4'0973   79–1654
ISBN 0–06–010436–8

80 81 82 83 10 9 8 7 6 5 4 3 2 1

This one is for my daughter Doré, whose sheer looming transcendence has filled my life with joy and infused it with meaning.

Contents

Preface

Rehabilitating America is for me as much a portrait of a certain present as a vision of a possible future. I have tried in writing this book to examine four of our most perplexing and paradoxical problems, those of ever-rising inflation, persistent poverty, increasingly burdensome government, and the growing longevity of our people, seeking within and among them some common thread I could unravel and pursue. I believe I have found one.

These four problems have proven remarkably resistant to the efforts we have made to date to control and manage them. Not the least of our difficulties has been that measures taken to solve one problem often exacerbate another. This "certain present" confronts us with painful choices, seeming to force us to choose between equally appalling alternatives. If we move aggressively against inflation, we risk increasing unemployment. When we try to reduce government expenditures, it appears that we must sacrifice the well-being of many of our poor and elderly citizens who need services provided by government to survive. The choices we face have been debated endlessly in government and the media. Perhaps nothing about all of this is more poignant than the frustration of the person in the street, caught between crosswinds and helpless to control their direction.

It would indeed be presumptuous of me to claim that the "thread" I believe I have found would solve these problems quickly and painlessly. It is not a panacea I have sought, but a place to begin. I have looked for some problem we can solve, one which contributes to each of the four other problems and at the same time forms a part of their solution. Despite these limitations, I suspect the reader will express considerable surprise at my choice of a thread and significant doubt about the importance of the issue and the likelihood that its resolution would have a potent impact upon the four problems I have identified.

This doubt surely will be strengthened when the reader sees the price tags for the steps proposed in this book. These five steps, taken together, will average about $22 billion a year for approximately ten years. And it will not be possible to pursue one step and ignore another; implementation of all five is required to make the approach successful. We can reduce our investment in any one or more of the five so long as we support all five, but the more we cut, the longer the process will take and the less likely its success becomes.

Can we afford to spend—on the federal, state, local, and private levels—as much as $22 billion annually? The answer, perhaps surprisingly, is not only that we can afford to, but that we literally cannot afford not to. The costs of *not* implementing these five steps may exceed *$150 billion each year.* These government and private expenditures, lost wages, and other costs will consume more than one thousand billion dollars, or $1 trillion, by 1990. And, unlike the expenses proposed here, these costs will not decline sharply after ten years, nor will they pay for themselves. Rather they will escalate in what will quickly become an uncontrollable spiral. Every working American will be supporting at least one other person in addition to his or her own dependents. For most of us, this will be an unaffordable future.

What, then, is the thread that links these four problems? It is the "problem of disability." We as a nation have failed to invest in the potential of our children, youth, adults, and elderly citizens who have physical, mental, and emotional disabilities. As a result, dependency among these people, who number in the tens of millions and whose number is constantly increasing, has become a major cause of inflation, a central factor in our country's poverty problem, one of the largest contributors to the annual increases in federal spending, and an important reason the "graying of America" has emerged as one of our most difficult social problems.

Inflation.[1] Dependency among disabled people now accounts for almost 9% of the nation's Gross National Product (GNP). Over the past decade, while inflation has grown so fast that the purchasing power of the dollar has been halved, dependency costs attributable to disability have risen much faster, feeding inflation at an alarming pace. Our investment on the federal, state, local, and private levels in dependency among disabled Americans now accounts for more money than does the national defense. If we were to call these costs a "budget," they would form the third largest budget in the world, after those of the United States and the Soviet Union. All of this can only mean that if we can somehow halt and then reverse the direction of spending on disability, we can make a significant impact on inflation.

Poverty.[2] Disability is a major cause of poverty, and poverty of disability. Of all families on welfare rolls, fully 20% are there because the head of the household is disabled. A member of a lower-class family is twice as likely in any given year to become disabled as is a member of a middle-class family. More than 60% of all poor families having at least a husband and a wife at home include a disabled adult. Almost half of the adult disabled population is at or near the poverty level. To alleviate and then eradicate poverty in our country, we must attack the problem of disability.

Government.[3] The largest, and fastest-growing, component of the federal budget is the so-called "uncontrollable" segment, that is, payments to individuals who are dependent upon and entitled to governmental aid. These costs are rising at a rate of 11% annually and have quadrupled over the past decade. Almost $40 billion of the total goes for disability benefits providing income-maintenance, medical-support, and related payments to disabled individuals. Five million such persons are on Social Security Disability Insurance, two million are on Supplemental Security Income, three million receive Medicaid benefits, and one million obtain food payments. These benefits for dependent disabled persons account for one out of every thirteen dollars in the federal budget. And it is exactly here that we can make perhaps our most impressive cuts. While not all disabled people can (or should) leave dependency rolls, many can. The combination of savings in the "uncontrollable" programs and increases in social-security and income taxes paid by the now-employed disabled individuals would be sufficient to slash the taxes of each and every American worker by several hundreds of dollars annually. The huge 1977 social-security tax hike, for example, might be partially rescinded: one-third of it was required to pay for anticipated disability benefits alone. This will happen only if we make sizable numbers of disabled people self-sufficient and independent. To do this, we must invest in their potential. But it is a sound investment by any measure.

Aging.[4] The emergence of "the four-generation society" imposes heavy burdens upon our nation precisely because we have not been able to find ways to reduce dependency among the old, one quarter of whom are disabled. Spending on the elderly now accounts for 25% of the entire federal budget. If present trends continue, spending on elderly citizens may triple within the next thirty years. Many old people now on dependency programs could work or contribute in other ways to society. Many others need not be placed in institutions, nursing homes, or other segregated and highly expensive settings, but could function within the community if we remove some of the architectural, transportation, and other barriers that now confront them, and if we find ways to use their talents and abilities more effectively. *These steps are in many respects the same as those we must take to make disabled people more independent:* we must make our job requirements truly work-related, we need to substitute ramps for stairs, we must make our transportation and housing programs fully accessible, and we need to alter our attitudes toward disabled and elderly persons, looking not so much at what they cannot do as at what they can, finding ways to benefit from what they have to contribute to society.

Disability, then, forms a part of each of the four problems and serves as a component for the solution of each. The "problem of disability" has become one of our most urgent national concerns. We are not accustomed to thinking of disability in these terms. Many of us have difficulty realizing that one out of every six of us, or thirty-six million, is disabled. Few of us know that by the year 2000, there will be one chronically ill, over-sixty-five, or disabled citizen for every able-bodied person in this country. These facts help explain why resolving the problem of disability can have such dramatic effects upon inflation, poverty, government expenditures, and the burdens of the four-generation society.

The task I have set for myself in this book is to envision and to describe an approach to the problems I have mentioned that will at once assist people who are disabled and elderly to achieve some measure of equality of opportunity in our society and at the same time constitute sound social policy for our nation as a whole. For just as I believe that America handicaps disabled people, and by so doing handicaps itself as well, so too do I believe that America can rehabilitate not only its citizens who are disabled but itself as well.

I must hasten to explain what I mean by that.

The problem of disability is, I have said, one that is rapidly assuming staggering proportions. This is a shock to many of us. Disability, when it has come to our attention at all, has generated feelings more akin to sympathy and concern than to determination and an urgent need for re-examination and change. What has always been seen as a separate, "special," and relatively minor problem is now understood by more and more of us as inextricably intertwined with other crises we face. We are just now beginning to see that neither this problem nor the others can be resolved without forever altering the ways we perceive people who are disabled.

Yet, and here is the twist, we are raising our consciousnesses to the problem of disability at precisely the moment when our capacity to cope with it is perceived to be markedly diminished. Rampant inflation has brought us crashing into an "era of limits," in which we understand as never before that problems may not yield quickly to massive infusions of funds, and in which we as a society appear to be tilting to the right in our expectations from government, looking to it less to expand in order to confront social problems than to reduce its burden upon us.

It would be perhaps the supreme irony if disabled people were to become the first victims of an inflation caused by the very programs and activities to which they were never granted real access and from which they have never benefited fully. To have come so close to a fighting chance at equality after a lifetime of segregation and exclusion would be bitter indeed for America's disabled citizens. As one put it recently: "Just when it's our turn to get a piece of the pie, people decide that we can no longer afford dessert."[5]

But that is wrong: We as a nation literally cannot afford not to have dessert. This is something almost no one understands: it is far more expensive to continue handicapping America than it would be to begin rehabilitating America. Keeping disabled people in dependency is costing us many times more than would helping them to independence. Put differently, *to "do nothing" now on the basis that our ability to respond to the problem is constrained by inflation is to feed that inflation and further reduce our capacity to solve the problem of disability.* And more, it would likely cripple our efforts to overcome poverty, big government, and the burden of increased longevity as well. It is an option we cannot choose. We must rehabilitate disabled people in order to rehabilitate America, and we must do it soon.

The surprise in all of this is that the future is a possible one: the problem of disability is a problem we can solve. There are five specific steps we can take, now, to rehabilitate America by rehabilitating her disabled citizens. And the $22 billion price tag for these steps is not an unreasonable amount. It is just $450 a year for each of the country's fifty million disabled and elderly citizens. The strategy proposed in this book will, I am convinced, help us accomplish both objectives so that they, in turn, may enhance each other. It is only by working toward both that we will reach either. For that is the paradoxical nature of the problem of disability: it can only be solved by transcending its conflicts.

Several people deserve my deepest thanks for stimulating me toward the ideas expressed in this book. Howard Rusk I must thank first. His vision of the possible future is much clearer than my own. Jack Duncan gave generously of his time that I might come to share his aspirations; he has taught me more than I can ever realize. Bob Butler helped me in many long and often-heated debates while we were both consultants to the U.S. House of Representatives Committee on Science and Technology, and it was in these discussions that many of the ideas found here first struggled to light. Monroe Berkowitz and his colleagues at Rutgers University provided indispensable statistical corroboration for many of the themes developed in this book. And throughout my work on disability, no one has been more supportive and insistent than Joe Owens. He contributed greatly to *Handicapping America* and even more meaningfully to this book.

I want to reserve special thanks for Prime Minister Menachem Begin of Israel and his wife Aliza. By their kind invitation, I was able to broaden my perspectives on the problem of disability greatly by comparing the approaches taken to its resolution in Israel and the United States. Israel has successfully rehabilitated fully 97% of its twenty thousand veterans with service-connected disabilities, and brought them back to work, so that they are now contributing members of Israeli society, imposing very little if any burden upon their fellow citizens. While commitment from the highest levels undoubtedly helped make this possible—Begin, for example, gave much of his $85,000 Nobel Peace Prize award for programs benefiting disabled people[6]—the Israeli example is nevertheless highly instructive for those of us in the United States.

REHABILITATING AMERICA

"I sense in our country a growing mood of withdrawal and isolationism, a retreat from obligations stated and unstated, a desire to redefine everything in terms that only serve the self rather than defining the self with a civic sense for others."

A. Bartlett Giamatti, President, Yale University,
addressing the Class of 1982

1 The Paradox of Costs

As America enters the 1980s, the restrictive attitudes toward social programming reflected in and instigated by California's "Proposition 13" tax revolt and its successors, a growing "conservative shift" in the population generally, and spiralling inflation combine to produce unprecedented pressure to "contain" and "manage" the problem of disability. The Congress and the administration are curtailing expenditures on programs serving disabled people in the belief that by so doing they are helping to curb inflation. State and municipal governments are lobbying hard in Washington against new federal initiatives requiring them to serve disabled people on the ground that they cannot afford new programs. And the American people increasingly are turning away from social concerns to self-fulfillment and leisure activities in what is being called the "Me Generation."[1]

There can be no question that, overall, Washington's policy is a sound one. Inflation ravages the very fabric of our society, debilitating our capacity to respond to our most pressing needs and forcing curtailment in many vital services and programs. Its conquest is of paramount importance. Certainly, our citizens who are disabled and elderly suffer much more than do other Americans from rising inflation and therefore have a great stake in the successful resolution of this continuing problem. Despite all of this, there is something seriously wrong with the approach being taken in the nation's capital and in state capitals throughout the country. This mistake lies at the very heart of the problem of disability and, by extension, at the core of the problems of inflation, poverty, big government, and increased longevity. For this reason, I want to address it immediately.

To begin, let me pose a rather rhetorical question: Do we, as a people, expect disabled persons to become taxpayers or are we generally content, or resigned, to their being tax-users? To state it differently: Do we as a nation see these people more as *able* than as *disabled,* as citizens expected to become self-sufficient and contributing members of society or as individuals needing continuing and even perpetual care? The question is a central one. And the answer is by no means self-evident.

Looking at our country's investment in disabled people, we find the answer: We usually regard these people as individuals requiring assistance, care, protection, and charity. Our answer bears a remarkable resemblance to that we would give to a similar question about elderly persons. Accordingly, we tend to "write off" the expenditures we make out of our income and social-security taxes for "entitlement" programs, that is, "uncontrollable" expenses. We see these as inevitable costs and concentrate our energy upon improving management and control of the programs, seeking more to eliminate fraud, duplication, and error than to question the very basis for these efforts. By contrast, we tend, again because of our perceptions, to study much more closely the "discretionary" or "controllable" costs allocated toward helping these people become more independent. When we cut our federal and state budgets, it is rarely to slash the uncontrollable costs; rather, we deplete already meager funds for educational and rehabilitation programs.

The essence of the argument I am trying to present is that by doing so we are crippling our ability to solve the very problems we think we are addressing. Persons who are disabled and many who are elderly are people with potential, ability, and productivity. These are people who could, and should, be self-sustaining. We cannot help them become so without increasing our investment in discretionary, controllable programs aimed at developing, nourishing, and refining that potential. In simpler terms, to save money we have to spend it.

This is the irony: It is only by increasing our investment in such programs as special education, rehabilitation, barrier removal, and research and technology that we can hope to make a meaningful dent in the huge costs incurred by our society because of dependence among disabled and elderly persons. We have not done so, and the results are unmistakable. They have helped lead to the present crises in inflation, poverty, big government, and longevity.

The Costs of Dependence

The 1977 social-security tax hikes were required, in large part, because the disability trust fund and old-age survivor's insurance programs were rapidly approaching bankruptcy. The new law makes the programs solvent for the next seventy-five years, but at a high cost. The price for every covered worker, ninety million of us, has already begun to be felt and will exert its pressure more and more through the mid-1980s.

Slightly less than one-tenth of the federal budget is now given over to disability. In fact, looking at the federal budget as a whole, now and over the foreseeable future, we find that "uncontrollable" expenses for disabled and elderly persons may account for almost half of all federal outlays before the century is over, while many of us are still working.

Even if we restrict ourselves to the present and limit our inquiry to disability alone, we find that we are talking about hundreds of billions of dollars annually. Today, America is spending ten dollars on dependence among disabled people for every dollar it expends upon programs helping them become independent. Few statistics so graphically portray the fact that our attitudes toward these people are oriented more toward dependence than independence—and are tragically mistaken.

Dependence-oriented programs include Social Security Disability Insurance (SSDI), Supplemental Security Income (SSI), and similar medical-payment and income-support efforts. These are programs that are entitlement in nature and that are contingent upon dependence; that is, disabled persons who are unable to work or engage in "substantial gainful activity" are entitled to benefits so long as they continue to be "unable to support themselves." The costs incurred in these programs, then, are costs we as a society bear because of dependence among disabled people. Direct-service programs, by contrast, are not entitlement in nature, but rather are goal-directed activities providing training and other services enabling disabled people to achieve independence. Prominent among these are special education and rehabilitation: both programs help disabled persons prepare for and obtain employment commensurate with their abilities and interests. And these are diverse indeed: such disabilities as deafness, blindness, cerebral palsy, paraplegia and quadriplegia, multiple sclerosis, epilepsy, learning disability, and many forms of mental retardation limit but do not preclude vocational potential. *In fact, we have found that anyone who is reasonably alert and has at least some movement, even if only in one limb, can be trained to work in competitive settings.* Disabled people are more able than they are disabled; the difference between those who become self-sufficient and those who do not is less a function of the severity of the disability than it is a reflection of the power and timeliness of the rehabilitation intervention. Yet our policies and programs continue to reflect the mistaken belief that they are unable to work and support themselves.

Consider, for example, the Carter administration's Fiscal Year 1980 Budget. While admitting that thirty-nine cents of every dollar in the federal budget was needed for entitlement and other benefit payments to individuals, the administration's "lean and austere" budget proposed little in the way of reduction in these uncontrollable items. Rather, it suggested decreases in real spending for rehabilitation, disability research, and other programs that would help remove disabled and many elderly persons from the dependence rolls. In following this path, the administration continued the pattern set by earlier administrations. Perhaps no one has shown this more clearly than Monroe

Berkowitz of Rutgers University, probably our most distinguished economist on disability issues.

What Berkowitz and his colleagues, notably Jeffrey Rubin, did was to compare dependence and independence costs over more than one decade. (While their use of these terms differs somewhat from my own, these divergences do not affect the essential validity of the argument.[2]) Taking into account federal, state, local, and private expenditures, they looked at income-maintenance, medical, and direct-service payments during the period 1967–75 and made projections for 1980. In 1967, federal, state, local, and private spending on dependence-oriented programs totalled $38.7 billion, while independence-oriented expenditures were less than $0.7 billion. The $39.4 billion total was 5% of the GNP for that year. By 1970, the total cost of these programs was $59.1 billion, or 6% of the GNP. Direct services (independence-oriented costs) were $1.2 billion, while transfer and medical payments incurred because of dependence were $57.9 billion. Three years later, in 1973, the total cost had reached $83 billion, or 6.5% of the GNP, with $80.8 billion allocated to dependence-oriented programs and $2.3 billion to direct services. In 1975, the total was $114 billion, or 7.9% of the GNP. The proportion expended on dependence had grown to $111 billion, while that given over to direct services was $3 billion. By 1980, assuming a moderate rate of inflation, Berkowitz and Rubin estimate the dependence total will be $210 billion. To grasp the magnitude of this sum, consider that it exceeds the total budget for 1980 of the entire U.S. Department of Health, Education, and Welfare (HEW), which was in turn the third largest budget in the world, after those of the United States and the Soviet Union.

These are staggering figures. They illustrate, first, that dependence among disabled people is a major factor in inflation. The dependence-oriented expenses grew at a rate much faster than that of inflation over the same period: between 1970 and 1975, for example, these costs almost doubled in current dollars and increased 40% in constant dollars. Second, we as a nation are spending enormous sums on income- and medical-support programs for disabled people but very little by comparison on direct-service programs which would help these persons move off dependence-oriented programs. Third, unless we alter direction dramatically and quickly, dependence among disabled people will continue to feed inflation at a dangerous pace, with no end to the spiral in sight.

This must mean that if we can control, and reverse, the direction of payments—if we can, that is, help disabled people become tax-payers rather than tax-users, thus contributing to the federal treasury and not withdrawing from it—we can significantly reduce inflation. To state it differently: If we inject increased support into direct-service programs such as special education and rehabilitation, we can help constrain expenditures on dependence, halting the spiral and then reversing it. Spending money on independence will save much more on dependence. This is why the paradoxical assertion that rehabilitating disabled people does not cost so much as it pays is true. This is a problem we can "solve by throwing money at it."

Disability and Poverty

Another, equally helpful, way to look at the problem of disability is to recognize that it is a problem closely linked with that of poverty in our country.

The onset of disability in a worker most often produces a traumatic loss in earning power. Fully three-fifths of disabled adults of working age are at or near the poverty level. The average annual "income" for disabled persons who are not married is $1,600; for married disabled individuals, the figure is $6,000. These totals include not only the earned income of the disabled person but also the contributions of others living in the household (notably those of nondisabled spouses in the case of married disabled individuals), insurance benefits, annuities, and income-maintenance monies.

On the other side of the coin is disability caused in part by poverty. Of course, it is not poverty itself but the conditions surrounding poverty that lead to disability. The rate of disability among blacks, for example, is double that among other races in our country. Of the seven million disabled children in school today, almost half are believed to come from inner-city families.

A closely related problem is that of unemployment. While we can consider this as a problem concerning those who are seeking work but cannot find it, it is much more realistic to perceive the problem more broadly as encompassing those who have given up looking for work. That is, many Americans, especially those confronted by immense barriers to employment, drop out of the labor force altogether. Because they have stopped looking for work, they are no longer counted as unemployed. Yet these are the people most likely to be in poverty.

When we examine disability and labor-force participation, we find, astonishingly, that an actual majority of disabled adults is not working. Of the fifteen million disabled Americans between the ages of sixteen and sixty-four who are not institutionalized, more than 7.7 million are either out of the labor force or unemployed. Most have given up looking for jobs. And they have done so because they cannot obtain the education they need for employment, cannot get job training in many fields, cannot secure transportation to and from work, cannot obtain access to places of work, and cannot find suitable places to live. Our failure to invest in these people and their potential has forced them into dependence programs. Among the more severely disabled, the proportion that is not working is nine out of ten. About 25% of all persons not in the labor force are disabled, and almost the same proportion holds for those in the labor force but unemployed.[3]

We can examine the problem further by looking at sources of income, marital status, age, race, and beneficiary status. Whereas nondisabled persons obtain almost all of their income from earnings, this is not true of disabled individuals. Almost two-thirds of the severely disabled people studied by the Social Security Administration in its most recent survey received public income-maintenance benefits, as did one-half of all disabled persons surveyed. Looking at the figures from a different perspective, we see that only one-half of all disabled persons and one-fourth of severely disabled individuals studied reported any earnings at all.

With respect to marital status, unmarried disabled men reported earnings in only three-fifths of the cases studied; among women who were not married, the proportion was less than two-fifths. Among those who were married, one would expect that a nondisabled spouse would go to work or work more following the onset of disability in the other spouse. In fact, this seldom occurred. Spouses, whether husbands or wives, were more likely to stay home to care for the disabled individual. This is particularly true of couples aged 35–44.[4] Reliance upon public income-maintenance funds, by contrast, increased with age: while 47% of severely disabled persons under age thirty-five received such funds, the proportion among those aged 55–64 was 71%. Black disabled persons were more likely than whites to receive public support and less likely to report earnings.

A Growing Burden

If the disability problem is being defined as a problem of costs, we have been focussing upon the wrong costs. The figures just presented illustrate that the overwhelming proportion of the costs associated with disability are costs incurred because of dependence among disabled persons—not costs related to services helping them become independent. Yet it is these independence-program costs that are being slashed, not the dependence-oriented expenses.

Investments in education and rehabilitation have barely kept pace with inflation, producing a levelling-off of actual spending power in these programs. In fact, one million out of the eight million children and youths in this country who are disabled are not even in school; rehabilitation programs have to decline services to eleven fully eligible persons for every one they can serve.[5] What has been the effect upon earnings (independence) and public income-maintenance payments (dependence) of this plateau?

If we look at two periods studied by the Social Security Administration (SSA), 1965 and 1971, we find that earnings accounted for less and public income maintenance for more of the income of disabled persons in 1971 than in 1965. In fact, a smaller proportion of disabled persons was employed in 1971 than in 1965. While some of the differences between the two periods may be accounted for by other factors, notably the prevailing economic conditions in the country as a whole, these can explain only some of the difference. Much of the effect is attributable to the inability of many disabled persons to secure the education and rehabilitation they required in order to find work.[6] More recent SSA figures confirm the trend.

That the burden of dependence upon our economy is growing is shown also by the Berkowitz & Rubin data discussed earlier. Strikingly, the Rutgers researchers find no increase in the number of disabled persons comparable to the huge increases in disability dependence expenditures incurred on the federal, state, local, and private levels. Thus the soaring costs cannot be attributed to increases in the disabled population or a general decline in the national health. What, then, explains the large increase in dependence expenditures?

I have already noted the lack of real growth in direct-service programs. This is certainly a factor, but it is an effect of a more basic cause: the perception of disabled people that characterizes us as a society. The difference between independence- and dependence-oriented expenditures is a fundamental one, and the way our country allocates its resources between them reveals a great deal about its expectations from disabled people. The evidence in the figures is that our society does not really believe that disabled people can become independent taxpaying citizens. This may be seen, as well, in the outcry over the anticipated costs for removing architectural and other barriers facing disabled people. Many college and university officials, for example, echoed Dr. A. G. Unklesbay, vice-president of the University of Missouri, when he complained that HEW's section 504 regulation requiring such removals would force many institutions "to prepare facilities that almost certainly will never be used."[7]

Closely related to this perception is the low visibility of the disabled population as a whole. Public policy toward women and members of racial minorities attracts far greater attention in America today than does policy toward disabled people. Perhaps it is because we as a society do not want to be reminded of it, but it seems to come as a shock for many people that the disabled population numbers thirty-six million and that fully 15% of all persons of working age are disabled. So long as our country does not appreciate the true size of this population, we will continue to be reluctant to allocate large proportions of our discretionary funds for its benefit.

A 1978 survey by Yankelovich, Skelly, and White, the respected opinion-research firm, revealed for the first time that some of these perceptions are changing. The findings are dramatic in their implications for our country's willingness to confront, at long last, the problem of disability.[8]

Support for "Special Efforts" and Advocacy

The Yankelovich survey was conducted in two phases as part of a larger series of studies. The first phase featured interviews with 2,224 members of the general public; the second, 149 "opinion leaders," including lawmakers, public-agency administrators, interest-group representatives, and other prominent figures.

The general-public sample was asked whether it supported "special efforts" on behalf of disabled people, minorities, women, and ex-convicts. The term "special efforts" may be interpreted to mean accessibility modifications for disabled people, affirmative action in employment, and similar steps. The survey was taken after more than eighteen months of press coverage of the anticipated costs of access for disabled people.

Fully 79% of the respondents answered yes when asked whether they supported special efforts on behalf of disabled people. This was almost double the proportion that responded affirmatively with respect to special efforts on behalf of the other groups studied. The results were:

Table 1. Attitudes toward "Special Efforts"

General Sample (N = 2234)

	Disabled People[a]	Minorities	Women	Ex-Convicts
YES	79%	44%	47%	38%
NO	14	49	46	45
DON'T KNOW	7	7	7	18

[a] The proportions held remarkably firm (± 2%) regardless of age, sex, race, economic status, education, and employment of the respondent.

Source: Yankelovich, Skelly, & White, 1978.

The findings with respect to special efforts on behalf of disabled people were almost identical among males and females, blacks and whites, young and old, poor and middle- or upper-class, low-educated and high-educated, and employed and unemployed.

The strength and scope of the support for special efforts for disabled people are surprising in light of the fiscal-expenditure and historical-attitude factors reviewed earlier. They are particularly startling coming as they do in the same summer that California's "Proposition 13" heralded a "tax revolt" which was widely interpreted to mean that more social spending was anathema to many Americans.

The results indicate that despite the fact that special efforts on behalf of disabled people are expected to be costly, almost eight Americans in every ten support such attempts. Disability rights may be one notable exception to the reported growing public aversion to social programming. If this is an accurate reading of these data, it is welcome news indeed.

Perhaps even more surprising was the endorsement of advocacy on behalf of disabled people found among the general public and opinion leaders. The general sample was asked to choose one of three statements describing advocacy: "Advocates for the handicapped are mostly asking for long-overdue changes"; "Advocates for the rights of the handicapped are sometimes unrealistic in their demands"; and "Neither." Seven in ten, or 71%, chose the first statement as most accurately matching their perceptions, while 25% chose the second, and 4% the third.

These results, in conjunction with the earlier data on special efforts, reveal that the members of the general public sampled in the survey believe that the barrier-removal and other activities that will be required on behalf of disabled people if these citizens are to achieve some measure of equality in our country are steps that should have been taken long ago and certainly must be taken now.

The opinion leaders surveyed were also asked a question about advocacy: "Do you see a need for more activist pressure by the handicapped?" The results, displayed in Table

2, are startling: two out of three did see such a need, while one of three did not. Among senators and congressmen, the proportions were better than seven out of every ten for more pressure, two of ten against, and almost one in ten undecided. Union leaders and interest-group representatives were even more emphatic in their support for such pressure. Only city officials, with 33% for more advocacy and 56% against, expressed reluctance to endorse civil-rights advocacy on behalf of disabled persons.

Table 2. Attitudes toward Advocacy

Opinion Leaders (N = 149)[a]

	Need More Pressure	Do Not Need More Pressure	Not Sure, NA
TOTAL	65%	29%	6%
Federal Legislators	72	20	8
Federal Agency Heads	68	32	—
Union Leaders	86	7	7
Interest Groups	83	11	6
State Legislators	67	25	8
City Officials	33	56	11

[a] "Do you see a need for more activist pressure by the handicapped?"

Source: Yankelovich, Skelly, & White, 1978.

These findings lend themselves to several possible interpretations. An obvious one is that the leaders, exposed as they are to heavy pressure from many special-interest groups, recognize that disabled people as a population have not yet brought their strength to bear upon public-policy issues to anything approaching the degree which their numbers would indicate. A second possible interpretation is that these decision makers desire more input from disabled people on how the problems this population faces might be solved. Independent evidence, reports from advocates on behalf of disabled people for example, indicates that there is a serious "information gap" between the recognition that "something has to be done" and knowledge of precisely what steps are likely to produce concrete results. A third possible explanation is that these leaders are seeking popular support for measures that they know will cost money and may prove controversial. This interpretation is illustrated in the remark attributed to then-President Lyndon Johnson in a meeting with Dr. Martin Luther King, Jr.: "You've convinced me. Now go out and bring pressure on me."

Whatever the basis for the opinion-leader survey results, the conclusion is inescapable that both the general public and key governmental and private-sector officials favor greater advocacy on behalf of disabled people. Equally vivid is the general public's willingness to support the kinds of special efforts these advocates will call for.

The Yankelovich survey is the first ever done on these kinds of questions by a national opinion-research firm. The data collected provide a foundation for beginning: we now know that if the problems disabled people face can be specified in manageable components, and ways to solve these problems found, it is entirely possible that these solutions will be implemented.

A Conflux of Paradoxes

We are faced, it seems, with a multitude of conflicting signals. On the one hand, America is unmistakably more conservative and cost conscious than it was in the early 1960s; on the other, the general public supports what it knows will be expensive changes benefiting disabled people. Similarly, the "Me Generation" is upon us, giving rise to the belief that "causes" are no longer popular; yet it is impossible to read the Yankelovich survey results without believing that here, at least, is a cause many Americans support. And while there is growing concern with the costs associated with barrier removal, comparatively little alarm has been expressed about the dependence-oriented expenditures, documented by Berkowitz and his colleagues. Which signals are we to trust and follow?

It would appear that the American public is responding more to its convictions than to complex statistical and financial evidence; that is, we may believe that it is "right" for disabled and elderly people to have an opportunity and that such chances have been denied them far too long. The American people, then, may be convinced that despite a general tightening in programming due to inflation, exceptions must be made. It is possible, too, that we are giving the general public too little credit for its sagacity. For, if the figures presented in this chapter tell us anything, it is that spending money to make disabled and elderly people increasingly independent is a wise investment, a decision entirely in keeping with a conservative economic and political philosophy. Thus, while the general public may not be aware of the staggering costs of dependency among disabled and elderly people, it may suspect as much, or at least understand that the country is better off with tax-payers living fully independent lives than with tax-users dependent upon others in the family and the community.

A Five-Point Plan

The question becomes, given these assumptions, what steps are required to bring about the desired result? What is it that we can do, as a country and as citizens of our communities, to help disabled and elderly people become more independent and self-sufficient?

The question is an important one for more reasons than may be immediately apparent. One distinguishing characteristic of the disability population is that it is an "open" one: anyone may join at any time. Disability is no respecter of wealth, age, sex, race, religion, or any other demographic factor. Thus, in posing this question, we are asking about a future that may become our own or that of someone close to us, as well as that of the thirty-six million Americans who are now disabled. And all of us can expect someday to become elderly. Second, the changes that will be needed for disabled and elderly people to enter the mainstream of society are in many instances changes that will benefit other persons as well. To choose just one example: The Transbus design for mass-transit buses, featuring wide doors, low floors, and ramps or lifts on the front doors, assists not only people who are disabled (about six million of whom cannot now use mass-transit bus transportation) but elderly individuals as well, as many as seven million of them, together with mothers pushing baby carriages, young children, men with temporarily sprained ankles, and shoppers burdened with heavy packages. In posing the question about what steps to take, we want to maximize such side effects as much as possible so that the investments we make will have the highest possible return for all of us. Third, and this must be stressed because of the propensity of so many of us to think of the disability problem as a "special" one, the steps we take must be steps that will help to solve the perplexing difficulties we face in the interaction of disability, inflation, poverty, big government, and longevity: we must bear in mind the need to do whatever we can to solve these problems together and simultaneously. Fourth, and finally, we must restrain ourselves to what is now within the realm of the possible: utopian solutions, however attractive, must be rejected. These steps must be practical moves we can make immediately.

Perhaps no one step will have so dramatic an impact as *expanding our research, development, and technology-transfer efforts* to increase our capacity to prevent, cure, and ameliorate the effects of age and disability. The potential inherent in these efforts is monumental. It is now possible, for example, to provide blind persons with machines that literally read aloud almost anything that is printed. The reverse of this technology, instrumentation that prints or "captions" auditory messages such as speech for deaf persons, is not immediately available but may be within our reach. And technology exists to permit a person so severely disabled that he or she can only speak, unable to move any other muscles voluntarily, to control almost any device or machine that operates electrically. Chapter 2, "Uncommon Sense," traces some approaches we can take to tap these research and technological developments, not only to remove the effects of disability but eventually to eradicate disability itself.

We must also continue *removing architectural, transportation, and communication barriers* facing disabled and elderly people. A vehicle exists in section 504 of the Rehabilitation Act of 1973, as amended, to accomplish much of the required barrier removal. Chapter 3, "The Barriers Come Tumbling Down," proposes specific alternatives we may choose in the areas of education, health services, housing, transportation, labor, social services, leisure and recreation, and other aspects of modern life, together with an analysis of the anticipated costs and benefits associated with these alternatives.

Third, we must mount a major effort to *train disabled and elderly people* not only how to overcome their disabilities but also how to tap their abilities so they may secure employment commensurate with their potential and interests. We can no longer be content with cost-of-living increases in our support for special education and rehabilitation. Rather, we as a nation must make a substantial investment in our disabled and elderly citizens by providing these direct-service programs with the support required to prepare disabled individuals for full employment. Chapter 4, "Reaching for Potential," presents an outline of how this might be accomplished.

At the same time, we must *reform the dependence-oriented programming* which now poses so many serious disincentives to employment for disabled and elderly people. Social Security Disability Insurance (SSDI), Supplemental Security Income (SSI), and other public-assistance and income-maintenance programs actually encourage disabled and elderly persons to rely upon federal assistance rather than to take a chance on competitive employment. Specific reforms are proposed in Chapter 5, "Dependence and Independence," reforms which are both realistic and likely to succeed in assisting many disabled and elderly persons to become self-sufficient. A major benefit associated with these reforms, if undertaken in conjunction with the other changes proposed, would be a dramatic reduction in dependence-oriented spending, with concomitant implications for inflation and federal expenditures on disability.

Finally, we must *make our communities "open" to and usable by disabled and elderly people.* This involves more than mere removal of barriers. It encompasses a multitude of often-small efforts that the average citizen can make in his or her own environment to make our cities and towns accessible. Chapter 6, "The Open Community," describes citizen advocacy on the local level, providing detailed suggestions and strategies.

The five points or steps are interrelated; they will succeed only if taken together. Reforming dependence-oriented programs to encourage employment, for example, is a pointless exercise unless we ensure that employment will be available and that the disabled or old person can get to and from the workplace. But the five steps offer a concrete series of initiatives that will help us to rehabilitate America by rehabilitating disabled people.

A Call to Conscience

The problem of disability has become a major problem of our times. It is interwoven intricately with the problems of poverty, inflation, big government, and increased longevity. We cannot escape it. But America has encountered "inescapable" problems before and occasionally has managed to avoid them, at least for considerable periods of time, sometimes by ignoring them, at other times by devising imaginative "solutions" that in fact merely submerged the underlying difficulty for another generation to face.

Objections to undertaking the steps proposed in this book are sure to be many; some of them have already been discussed. They are not dissimilar, though, to those faced, in another decade, by proponents of racial equality.

In 1963, Martin Luther King referred metaphorically to the "costs" confronting black people, costs disabled people encounter literally. In his "I Have a Dream" speech, King responded to these objections in words that I, too, might adopt:

> In a sense we have come to our nation's Capital to cash a check. When the architects of our republic wrote the magnificent words of the Constitution and the Declaration of Independence, they were signing a promissory note to which every American was to fall heir. This note was a promise that all men would be guaranteed the unalienable rights of life, liberty, and the pursuit of happiness.
>
> It is obvious today that America has defaulted on this promissory note insofar as her citizens of color are concerned. Instead of honoring this sacred obligation, America has given the Negro people a bad check; a check which has come back marked "insufficient funds." But we refuse to believe that the bank of justice is bankrupt. We refuse to believe that there are insufficient funds in the great vaults of opportunity of this nation. So we have come to cash this check—a check that will give us upon demand the riches of freedom and the security of justice.

So my final argument is one of equity: Will America respond to disabled and elderly people that there are "insufficient funds"—that there is no "dessert"—or will America begin to rehabilitate these people and, by so doing, rehabilitate itself?

I have talked in this chapter of inflation, poverty, and unemployment. And I have spoken of potential, a potential for disabled and elderly people and a potential for the country as a whole. It is to the tension between poverty and potential that this book is directed. I do not pretend to have all the answers, but I do hope to raise some of the right questions.

It will be up to each of us to answer these questions. I can envision two possible futures: one in which we choose to rehabilitate disabled people, thereby rehabilitating America, and another in which we do not. The Supreme Court, in its *Papachristou* decision, has enunciated the former much more vividly than can I: we, and disabled and elderly Americans in particular, will enjoy "independence and self-confidence, the feeling of creativity, . . . lives of high spirits, rather than hushed, suffocating silence."[9] And if we do not meet the challenge, Langston Hughes has said it best: "See what happens to a raisin in the sun, and a dream deferred too long."

"We have added years to life and now it is our responsibility to add life to years."

George Morris Piersol[1]

2 Uncommon Sense

Recent advances in the application of space-age technology and in basic and applied research have brought us to the very brink of an unprecedented breakthrough in the prevention, cure, and amelioration of disability in our country. For the first time, we can speak expectantly not only of helping disabled people to "overcome" their impairments but of eventually eradicating these limitations themselves. We are poised now for the exhilarating moment when we will be able to regenerate severed spinal cords and other impaired functions. These tantalizing possibilities may also help elderly people become more capable of leading productive and satisfying lives. And spin-offs of the space program offer us through technology transfer the prospect of mechanical devices enabling disabled people to do what was never before possible—to see despite blindness, move despite paralysis, and hear despite deafness. Common sense tells us this is impossible. But research is nothing if not uncommon sense.

All of this is not to say that the breakthrough will emerge of its own power, without major alterations and investments of financial and human resources. It is not to say that the changes will come without reverberations that challenge the very fabric of our ethical and cultural beliefs and institutions. And it is not to say that all of the promises that now appear so bright will be kept. But it is to say, and this is important, that for the first time in our nation's history we can begin to think of disability not so much as a devastatingly permanent condition but increasingly as a perhaps, just perhaps, temporary hurdle that can be grasped and swept aside.

The magnitude of the potential contrasts vividly with the paucity of our nation's investment in the work that has brought us to this moment. We are spending one dollar per disabled citizen per year on rehabilitation research and development (R&D). The federal commitment, by far the largest share of R&D expenditures, is only $30 million annually; as a percentage of all federal health-related expenditures, it is only 0.026%.[2] Compared with the total for all public and private research and development in health-related fields, spending on disability R&D is less than one percent. Equally discouraging, it is precisely this modest investment that is most likely to be slashed by a cost-conscious society.

It is difficult to understand, or to justify, the lack of investment in research and technology when the potential for disabled individuals, for the economy, and for the nation is so vast. Straining a bit, we may speculate that we as a people do not really believe that the efforts will yield tangible results. Or possibly the fact that such potential is within our grasp simply is not known except among a few researchers and knowledgeable insiders. And it may be that restraints upon disability R&D are largely a function of restricted investments in research generally. Whatever the reasons and whatever their past validity, they just will not wash now. A major national commitment to disability research and technology is perhaps the single most exciting step we can take to solve the problem of disability in our country today.

Let us review the state-of-the-art in research and technology by considering the recent developments and some protocols for future activity, first looking at the specific disability areas separately and then stepping back to perceive the overall picture that emerges and to address some of the medical, technical, and ethical questions that remain.

Spinal-Cord Injury[3]

More than half a million Americans have severed spinal cords, with ten thousand new cases being added annually. The bulk of the injuries occur in automobile accidents, in falls while skiing or sky diving, and in contact sports such as football and soccer. It is one of the most dramatic and severe of all disabilities because of the immediate, traumatic, and total impact upon everything the individual tries to do—and because the injury is so small and localized yet complete in its effect. Damage in the spinal cord may produce paraplegia, an inability to control the movements of the lower extremities of the body, or quadriplegia, in which the upper extremities are also affected. It can turn a healthy fullback who, one moment, is crashing off tackle for a touchdown into a youth who, the next moment, is paralyzed from the neck down.

The financial repercussions are almost as devastating. Medical rehabilitation and training at centers such as Baylor University's Texas Institute of Rehabilitation and Research may cost as much as $40,000.[4] Even at that price, rehabilitation is cost effective because institutionalization and lifelong medical-care costs, together with expenses to the individual and the family in lost income and other costs, are much higher.

Dr. Howard A. Rusk, testifying before Congress, explains it this way:

We spend that much money because we cannot afford not to. The answer is simple. The average age of our quadriplegics at the Institute [of Rehabilitation Medicine, New York University Medical Center, in New York City] is twenty years. Our followup studies have shown that if these patients follow the simple rules that they have been taught on prevention of bed sores, kidney complications, skin care, et cetera, their expectancy is within two years of normal. This means that the life expectancy of these young people is approximately 50 years. If you do nothing for these patients except keep them in bed with routine care in a nursing home, the average cost in the New York area including part-time attendance which is necessary, really, to keep them alive, the cost is at least $15,000 a year. The arithmetic is simple: $15,000 times 50 is $750,000. However, if you stop there you have not thought the problem through. If these costs are compounded as in a savings bank, the cost would be over $3 million during the life expectancy that someone would have to pay, and that "someone" would be us, the taxpayers. (Why not let their families look after them?) That would mean two people out of the work force indefinitely, and the cost would be more than the dollar figure.

Two R&D developments—one in medical research and one in technology transfer—appear especially promising. Researchers at Georgetown University reported on November 6, 1978, that they have met with "encouraging initial success" in repairing damaged spinal cords. The work of Carl Kao and his colleagues on regeneration of surgically damaged spinal cords in dogs is the first solid indication that spinal-cord injuries are reversible. While application of the techniques to human beings awaits further research, Kao's findings are remarkable in that they reveal that the nerve fibers in the spinal cord do grow after the cord has been crushed: "The axons were trying to come down," Kao told Washington *Post* reporter B. D. Colen, "and they have lots of power to come down, but when they get to the end [of the break] the insulation of the nerve in the spinal cord is so sticky and fragile, it's just like a sleeve. There's no way the axon can come out unless it explodes, and when it explodes it explodes itself. And it has enzymes that destroy the entire area. So any attempts at regeneration always end in self-destruction."[5] This is why, prior to Kao's breakthrough, nerve grafting never succeeded.

What Kao did was to discover that by waiting one week after the injury he could insert nerve cells into the severed spinal cord and have the graft "hold." Five of the forty dogs he studied walked after the operation, and many of the other dogs exhibited evidence that the operation was at least partially effective. It was the first successful attempt at spinal-cord regeneration ever reported. If further work on cats and other animals is equally promising, the implications for human spinal-cord repair are huge. Even the one-week waiting period, if it applies to human beings as to dogs, is propitious because it allows doctors sufficient time to identify potential patients and prepare them for surgery.

Technology-transfer developments of great promise are currently being studied. One of the most exciting is the electronic wheelchair designed at New York University which enables a severely disabled individual to control virtually anything in his environment that operates electrically by means of a computer-assisted, voice-controlled word bank. The device currently has an eighty-word capacity, programmable in any language. An individual who is completely paralyzed but can speak merely enunciates his or her commands ("TV on," "Change channel," et cetera) and the chair does the rest. Because it is a prototype, one of only a few in the country, the cost of the chair is very high (about $35,000). Nevertheless, with large-scale production, it may prove markedly cost effective. Consider, for example, that it permits a severely disabled person to do many things he or she previously had to depend upon an attendant to perform. At the current hourly rate for attendants, $3 an hour or $24 for an eight-hour day, it is theoretically possible for such a chair to amortize, or "pay for," itself within one or, at the most, two years. And the employment opportunities opened because the chair may permit operation of electrically controlled devices, such as computer terminals, accelerate the potential return on investment considerably. The human benefits, while less tangible, are great in that the person is much less dependent upon others for performance of many routine daily tasks.[6]

Equally important are safety measures such as air bags and occupational and industrial procedures that may prevent many accidents which now produce spinal-cord injuries. The National Safety Council has estimated, for example, that 1.9 million persons have been disabled in automobile accidents and 2.2 million in industrial accidents in this century.

Other research and technology developments may help to alleviate pressure sores, which are a major source of difficulty for many spinal-cord-injured persons and a significant cause of time lost from work for those who are employed. Advances in orthotics, prosthetics, and adaptive equipment, particularly in enabling an individual to move his or her arms and legs, drive a car with hand controls, climb unramped stairs in a wheelchair, and dial a telephone, are exciting, although manpower shortages in this area are severe and worsening annually.

Many quadriplegic individuals have difficulty sustaining the breathing process because of the injury. It is necessary for them to spend considerable amounts of time, perhaps as much as eight hours daily, using an iron lung. Researchers at Brown University and other centers are experimenting with implantable "booster lungs" which are made of Teflon. While considerable research remains, particularly in testing the devices in animals such as sheep, the possibilities for increasing the mobility and independence of severely disabled individuals are great. Pierre Galletti, professor of medical science at Brown and a past president of the American Society for Artificial Internal Organs, is a pioneer in this area. He expects the lung to be especially helpful for persons with emphysema and other chronic lung diseases.

Probably the largest practical problem in spinal-cord-injury research is the field's inability to stimulate production of devices which have been designed and developed through rehabilitation engineering. A large number of prototypes are "on the shelf," many of which could contribute significantly to rehabilitation of spinal-cord-injured persons, but the production and distribution capabilities required for large-scale use are lacking. I shall return to this problem, which characterizes research and technology in other disability areas as well, in the later discussion of obstacles to application of R&D findings.

Blindness

An estimated 1.7 million Americans have severe visual impairments, of whom about one-half million are legally blind. Each year, thirty thousand persons lose their sight through accidents and illness. Almost half of all blind individuals are sixty-five years of age or older. Startlingly, however, blindness occurs much more frequently among poor people than among those of the middle and upper classes. For families with incomes under $2,000 annually, the rate of blindness is 12.3 per 1000 persons, compared to 1.59 per 1000 for families with incomes over $7,000. Malnutrition and poor medical care are two important reasons. These figures offer powerful evidence of the close relationship between poverty and disability.

Research and technology in the area of blindness have focussed largely upon communication and mobility, as these are the two greatest needs expressed by blind individuals. Innovations in braille writing (including "paperless braille," which uses magnetic tape to store materials which otherwise would be too bulky for storage and retrieval systems), electronic canes (including a "laser cane" which detects obstacles in the user's path), and other areas are exciting. Despite ten years of basic research, however, we are no closer than we ever were to implants into the visual cortex allowing blind persons to see, largely because of safety and performance questions. A recent development called the Kurzweil Reading Machine, though, holds tremendous potential for rehabilitating blind persons. Because, unlike many of the developments described in this chapter, the machine is already available, albeit in small numbers, it will be described at some length.

The Kurzweil Reading Machine is a fully automatic reader which scans a page, "recognizes" the words on it, and "reads" them out in a synthetic "voice." The device consists of three parts. The Reading Unit, on which the printed material is placed, is about the size of an electric typewriter. The Electronic Control Unit, about two cubic feet in size, contains a minicomputer and other special-purpose electronics. The Control Box, about the size of a desk calculator, contains the on/off and other controls.

The machine can read up to two hundred words per minute. The user can direct the machine to skim text rapidly or to read one word at a time; the machine will even spell out words upon demand. The processes involved are readily explained. A small electronic camera moves beneath the glass plate, converting the printed image into an electronic image which is then transmitted to the minicomputer in the Electronic Control Unit. The computer analyzes the electronic image to locate the letters, to recognize them, and to compute the sequence of speech sounds required to "say" the words. Special synthesizer circuits then produce the artificial speech enabling the blind person to hear what the machine is reading. For persons who are deaf as well as blind, attachment of a braille printer to the machine is feasible for braille output.

The reading machine was developed during five years of preliminary investigation, two years of prototype design, and another two years of further development. The first models marketed carried a price tag of $50,000, but the current version sells for about $20,000. While high, the cost is reasonable with respect to purchase by rehabilitation facilities and by schools and colleges for student use. Consider, for example, the possible applications of this machine for a college subject to the section 504 regulation issued by the Department of Health, Education, and Welfare requiring accessibility for blind as well as for other disabled students. Readers for blind students may cost the university as much as three or four dollars per hour per student, while relatively few materials are available in braille. Installation of a reading machine in the college library thus becomes potentially cost effective, while at the same time increasing the independence of the blind student, a not insignificant benefit.

The Kurzweil is not the only reading machine currently available. The Optacon, for example, is much less expensive (about $3,000) and is more generally available, with five thousand in existence. This machine copies into tactile form whatever image is presented to its camera. Unlike the Kurzweil, the Optacon is capable of reading nonverbal information, including electronic displays and graphs. It is slow, however, capable of reading between thirty and sixty words a minute, or one-tenth normal reading speed for sighted persons, and is difficult to use for persons whose tactile sensitivity is limited. It is, however, somewhat more adaptable than the Kurzweil to specialized vocational uses because its application is not limited to a restricted word-bank capability.

Mobility-aid R&D has been less successful, largely because of the unreliability of pilot-model devices, impracticability of some of the techniques, and unwillingness of blind individuals to undergo long training periods learning to use devices which are of limited assistance to them. No single device has reached more than five hundred blind persons and most have helped much fewer.

Researchers at the University of Utah in Salt Lake City and Columbia University in New York City are experimenting with electrical stimulation of the visual cortex through implanted electrodes. The technique bypasses the eye and the optic nerve, where lesions causing blindness are most common. While preliminary results are promising—volunteers who are blind report "seeing" light and other images—a great deal of work remains. William Dobelle, at Columbia's Division of Artificial Organs, is cautiously optimistic. In order for actual artificial sight to occur, he says, the blind individual would have to have a miniature television camera in his or her glasses or embedded in a glass eye, a minicomputer to convert the TV image into electrical stimuli that would be comprehensible to the brain, and electrodes attached to virtually every area of the brain specialized for sight. No such system has been developed, nor is there any assurance yet that it would work.

The reading machines, however, if given wide distribution and if improved over the current state-of-the-art, hold immediate and enormous potential for blind individuals. The impact upon vocational opportunities alone is vast. So, too, is the very meaningful everyday reduction in dependence upon sighted persons for reading mail, paying bills, and similar tasks.

Deafness

Hearing impairment is the single most prevalent chronic physical disability in the United States, with 6.6% of the population having some degree of hearing loss. About 1.4 million Americans are deaf, of whom almost one-half million became deaf early in life. Improvements in hearing-aid technology is important for the larger group of hearing-impaired individuals, but of little potential relevance for those who are deaf.

The teletypewriter (TTY) enables a deaf person to communicate over the telephone with others having similar devices. The machine works through an acoustic coupler which translates auditory messages into electronic impulses which activate a keyboard. The older TTYs have hard-copy printouts, while some of the newer devices do not. Costs range from $200 to almost $1,000, with the newer machines lightweight and fully portable. In large part because of the costs of the machines, fewer than 1% of all deaf persons in the United States own a TTY.

Telephone systems which can transmit both picture and sound are technically feasible and in fact exist. The Picture-phone developed by the Bell System is in use at the National Technical Institute for the Deaf (NTID) in Rochester. A combination television and telephone, it enables the two callers to see as well as hear each other. Mass production of the machine, however, has been terminated by the telephone company because the signals cannot be sent over traditional telephone wires; the larger cables that would be required would be expensive to install, and, according to the company, the utilization of the machine by the general public would not be widespread enough to justify these costs.

One other device enabling deaf people to use the telephone has been in existence since 1965 but has not caught on. This is the Electrowriter, which reproduces images with a stylus upon special paper. Like the TTY and the Picturephone, the device can only be used when both callers have the machine.

With respect to television, research and technology developments over the past few years have led to dramatic new possibilities for deaf people. "Captioning" of television is currently being done on selected programming telecast by the Public Broadcasting System (PBS), notably the "ABC Evening News" rebroadcast captioned by WGBH-TV in Boston each weekday evening. These captions are visible to all viewers, not only those who are deaf. By contrast, "closed captions," which use what is called "Line 21" on the television signal, are visible only to persons who purchase a decoding device or "black box." PBS recently began captioning many of its prime-time programming with closed captions in anticipation of the development and mass marketing of the decoder, now expected to cost between $200 and $300 each.

Both open and closed captioning require considerable "lead time" during which professional captioners prepare the captions. "Real-time" captioning, in which simultaneous written and auditory messages are transmitted, is not yet feasible. The technology is roughly the obverse of that developed in the Kurzweil Reading Machine for blind persons; what is needed for deaf people is a machine that prints what it hears rather than says what is sees. Still, there appears to be no compelling reason why a wordbank could not be developed and the necessary computer programming done, so that auditory messages might be "recognized" and printed versions produced. The implications of real-time captioning for deaf persons would be enormous, opening up tremendous employment opportunities and enabling deaf individuals previously deprived of entertainment through television, radio, theatre, and other media to enjoy the programming and information hearing persons take for granted.

Amputation

About one million Americans lack one or more limbs or extremities, while 2.5 million have impaired upper limbs and 7.4 million have impaired lower limbs. For many of these persons, orthotics and prosthetics are essential for daily living. Advances in prosthetic design, notably for greater comfort and lighter weight (through, for example, molded propylene rather than metal braces), artificial limbs, joint replacement, and mobility aids have been considerable in recent years. An indication of the great need in this area is the fact that the annual cost associated with pressure sores, including medical and lost-wages expenses, is $440 million. Patient costs related to failed implants and joint-replacement efforts are believed to be $80 million annually. The National Center for Health Statistics estimates that there are more than 2,000,000 orthopedic operations annually, and that there are in permanent use among the general population 2,500,000 special shoes, 2,000,000 canes, 500,000 crutches, 500,000 wheelchairs, 250,000 lower-limb orthoses, 800,000 other orthoses, and 172,000 prostheses.

Perhaps the greatest single area where research is needed is in pressure-sore management. The impact upon the lives of those affected is enormous, yet the basic research required to understand how tissue responds to pressure, and how to minimize adverse reactions, has yet to be done. The problem relates to wheelchair cushions, adapted footwear, bed mattresses, and other instances in which mechanical devices press upon tissue.

Some exciting research, much of it in the Soviet Union, is helping us understand why limb regeneration occurs in salamanders and newts but not in humans. N. Polezhayev, a professor at the Institute of Developmental Biology in Moscow, has regenerated limbs in newly born opossums and rats in precedent-shattering research and has predicted that similar regeneration may be possible in humans. Writing in the magazine *Science,* however, Arnold Caplan and Charles Ordahl suggest that a "switching off" process occurs in which cells which at one point in the organism's development might become any one of a number of organ or muscle tissues gradually "specialize" and lose their undifferentiated character. Caplan, of the Developmental Biology Center of Case Western Reserve University in Cleveland, and Ordahl, of Temple Medical School in Philadelphia, contend that this process would explain why regeneration may occur in newborns but not in older organisms. If they are correct, the implications of Polezhayev's work are severely limited. Still, there is a possibility that some work, such as recombinant DNA research, might yield up the undifferentiated-character potential even from mature cells, permitting cell regeneration to occur.[7]

We may not need to wait that long, however. Donald Lyman, director of the polymer implant center at the University of Utah, is investigating the use of synthesized implant surfaces under a grant from the National Institute of General Medical Sciences. The special surfaces permit only selected kinds of cells to "stick" to them, serving as scaffolding for their growth; long after the implant disintegrates, the regenerated cells would continue to grow. Lyman is particularly excited about the potential of polymer surfaces to reconnect severed nerves so the gaps will be bridged. The "cuff" would stimulate nerve growth while also facilitating growth of the cells that support the nerves. "Then," he told Maya Pines, "if you could get nerve signals through these cuffs, as we are attempting to do in the lab across gaps of one centimeter, you could repair different types of nerve loss and paralysis."

Lyman's colleague Stephen Jacobsen, director of the university's Projects and Design Laboratory, has developed an artificial arm that operates much as real arms do—and that an individual can control through the normal mind-arm voluntary-muscle processes. Studying the functions of each muscle in the arm, he and his assistants designed what they call a "Utah arm" that reproduces these functions. A microcomputer processes signals from the shoulder, allocating appropriate amounts of energy to miniature motors in the arm, while an artificial hand capable of grasping objects and lifting fifty-pound weights, is controlled by the motors. Jacobsen expects to test his prototype arm under actual living conditions and then to develop more sophisticated models which can do even more.

Speech Impairment

Approximately two million Americans have minor to severe impairments in speech, of whom almost two hundred thousand are limited in the amount and kind of work they can do because of these speech impediments. Research and technology in this area have concentrated upon design of devices which enable those who cannot talk to communicate with others and upon the development of voice-amplification and speech-training equipment.

An experimental microcomputer-based keyboard system developed by Bell Laboratories and the Telephone Pioneers of America permits a disabled person to compose messages by pressing large buttons on a special, oversized portable keyboard. The keyboard is coupled to a microcomputer and to a TV set and page printer. The message typed appears immediately upon the screen and, if desired, a printed copy is also produced. To reduce the amount of typing required, the computer stores abbreviations for words, word endings, and phrases, so that, for example, "GH" would produce a message reading, "I want to go home now." Bell Laboratories has preprogrammed a standard list of such abbreviations. The machine has important implications not only for speech-impaired individuals but also for those who are severely cerebral palsied or deaf and who are limited in oral communication.

Other devices produce synthesized speech or printed outputs. Input is usually alphabetic, although the newer machines will accept selections of whole words or phrases. No currently available system offers both printed and vocalized output. None are completely portable. Other areas in which improvements are needed include development of a device which would clarify or amplify speech so as to make it better understood. At Carnegie-Mellon University, a system is now being developed which has a one-thousand-word capability and which can, within certain semantic limits, comprehend about 95% of what is spoken. Subjecting the voice signal to selective bandpass filtering, frequency shifting, and other techniques may improve intelligibility.

Although most of these machines are at the prototype stage of development, they represent a significant advance over the standard keyboard-and-pointer technology which has been the mainstay for speech-impaired individuals. Other promising devices enable speech pathologists to show their clients the results of speech training, offering a kind of biofeedback reinforcement for improvements in speech output.

Mental Retardation

Research into mental retardation, much of it supported by the Kennedy family, has produced dramatic gains in our understanding of the causes of retardation—and has led the National Association for Retarded Citizens to speak hopefully of a possible cure.[8] Amniocentesis, the surgical insertion of a hollow needle through the abdominal wall and uterus of a pregnant woman to obtain amniotic fluid, enables detection of chromosomal abnormalities, including evidence of retardation. Its use, however, has generated controversy, particularly with respect to the ethical implications of abortion.

Other developments have been promising, as well, espe-

cially research showing that persons who are retarded may
be trained to perform work thought until very recently
to be impossible for them. By breaking tasks down into
manageable components and then teaching these subtasks
in carefully sequential and consecutively more complex
steps, it is possible to prepare educable retarded individuals for paid employment in the community as well as in
sheltered workshops and other restricted settings. We have
also learned that retarded persons can perform better than
normally intelligent individuals on highly repetitive, assem-
bly-line jobs. The obstacles remaining are less research
in nature than utilization and application in scope; e.g.,
convincing employers to hire retarded workers.

A Protocol for Progress

As promising as the recent developments in research and
technology are, realizing the potential will require a number of marked changes in the structure and funding patterns of R&D. In what follows, I have tried to outline what
some of these changes might be. Many of the ideas which
appear below were developed by the Panel on Research
Programs to Aid the Handicapped of the U.S. House of
Representatives Committee on Science and Technology
in 1977 and 1978. Others were suggested by the National
Academy of Sciences, especially in its report on "Science
and Technology in the Service of the Physically Handicapped," which was published in 1976. Finally, a series
of reports entitled "Human Rehabilitation Techniques,"
prepared for the National Science Foundation by Texas
Tech University, and a symposium convened by the Ameri-

can Association for the Advancement of Science in 1978, called "Science, Technology, and the Handicapped," were also helpful.

1. *Expand Federal Support for Disability R&D.* The present economic investment is much too nominal for the nation to meet its commitment to disabled people. Spending on disability, including all devices, systems, and research, averages just $2.92 per disabled person per year; the investment in research is only $1 per person per year. P.L. 95–602, the Rehabilitation, Comprehensive Services, and Developmental Disabilities Amendments of 1978, establishes a new National Institute of Handicapped Research which is to coordinate federal research on the prevention, cure, and rehabilitation of disability.

2. *Improve Coordination of Research Projects.* There is little sharing of information between governmental and private sources of research funding, and even between different governmental agencies. The quality of research can be improved markedly by enhancing dissemination of findings, sharing of knowledge, and coordination of resources. The need is especially critical with respect to access to R&D progress in other nations.

3. *Offer Governmental Underwriting of Technology.* Federal guarantees of a market for certain devices could prove to be the single most beneficial step we can take. Consider, for example, the implications for reducing the costs of these items. The Kurzweil Reading Machine now costs $20,000. If the federal government were to guarantee purchase of 250,000 of these machines, the company could market them at perhaps $450 each. Similarly, teletypewriters for deaf people (TTYs) could be sold for as little as

$25 apiece, while "black boxes" enabling deaf persons to receive closed captions on their television sets might cost as little as $20.

Other alternatives are also available. In Great Britain, for example, the government pays two-thirds of the cost of devices for blind persons, while the blind individual pays the balance. American health-care insurers such as Medicare and Medicaid generally do not pay for such devices but will pay for things that are done to the body or attached in or to the body; expansion of coverage to include engineering and other assistive devices would yield important benefits for many disabled individuals who could not otherwise afford the aids.

Regardless of the approach taken, ensuring a market is of enormous importance. Few private research and development institutes have production capabilities, and are therefore only able to produce prototypes. Private companies often are reluctant to make and distribute such devices in the absence of a large market and assurances that the target population is both able and willing to purchase the devices. The problem then becomes one of developing "on-the-shelf" technology which never reaches its intended audience. The difficulty is particularly acute with respect to low-volume products such as the NYU electronic wheelchair, where high initial cost combines with low potential-market size to discourage virtually any production and distribution effort.

4. Provide a Better Balance between Basic and Applied Research. The tendency in the recent past has been for applied research to be much better supported because of anticipated rapid "payoff" and because of restricted support for basic research generally. This has happened, for example, with pressure-sore research and the resulting lack of progress has been disastrous. The evidence is compelling in this as in a number of other areas that the answers are less likely to be found through engineering and technology than through basic research.

Similarly, it is only through basic research that we will be able to develop surgical bypasses for damaged optical and cortical nerves. In many instances of deafness, for example, the lesion does not exist in the ear itself but in the VIII nerve; if a way were to be found to bypass that nerve and to join the ear with the brain in some other way, hearing could be restored. And basic research offers our only hope for surgical regeneration of spinal-cord injury and other severe disabilities.

5. *Focus As Much on Low Technology As on High.* Our nation has become fascinated with high technology in which very sophisticated devices and techniques are applied to the solution of complex but rare problems. We have tended to neglect the more mundane, but more widely applicable, low technology. There is a wide gap between the demands of disabled consumers for low-cost, simple devices they can use immediately and the availability of funding for such technology. Similarly, the focus on high technology has tended to obscure the problem facing many disabled people of obtaining repairs for devices they already have.

6. *Develop Low-Cost Solutions to Problems of Barrier-Free Design.* While section 504 of the Rehabilitation Act of 1973, as amended, requires the removal of architectural, communication, transportation, and other barriers, insufficient knowledge exists on how these barriers may be removed without incurring high costs. The "knowledge gap" in this

area is a major impediment to mainstreaming disabled people into the community.

7. *Include Disability Questions on the U.S. Census.* Perhaps the greatest single obstacle facing the entire research, development, technology, and training effort on behalf of disabled people is lack of information on the size of the population and its characteristics. The census never has included questions designed to solve this problem, although the 1970 census did contain a small (5% sample) probe on disability. Our knowledge of the needs of this population is far from satisfactory, based as it is upon limited, special-purpose surveys and studies such as those conducted by the Social Security Administration. While the Census Bureau announced it would include at least one disability question in the 1980 decennial study, indications are increasing that this effort will not be expanded, largely because of difficulties in defining the term "disability" and in obtaining reliable data about prevalence and incidence.

It is difficult to overemphasize the importance of a sound statistical base. If we knew how many people have what disabilities, we could allocate scarce resources with much greater impact than is now possible. Similarly, our research and development efforts could be targeted with much greater precision. We would know to what extent our education and rehabilitation programs are serving their intended purposes—and exactly where, and with whom, they are not. Armed with this information, we would be able to institute changes in our service-delivery patterns and techniques so as to ensure that those with the most severe problems are served.

8. *Expand Consumer Involvement in R&D.* The tendency

to this point has been for disabled people, the intended consumers of R&D products, to be involved only at the very end of the development process, rather than at its outset. Only those who are themselves disabled know what it is that they need, what kinds of devices they will actually accept for daily use, and how much they can afford to pay (or are willing to pay) for the products of R&D. And the evidence is unmistakable that early involvement of consumers saves large amounts of time and money in designing products and stating research problems. This holds from planning and policy development to actual implementation or use of research and technology results.

9. Provide Tax Deductions for Adaptive Equipment. At present, only those devices which are medically prescribed or needed for health maintenance may be deducted on income tax returns. The inequity of this approach is readily appreciated when the costs of being disabled are computed. Inclusion of nonmedically related devices and aids as deductible items would likely provoke purchase of such devices, thus stimulating the industry considerably and producing, in turn, greater investments in R&D.

10. Develop and Enforce Standards for Equipment. In far too many cases, disability aids and devices are not regulated. Many of the companies producing these devices are small ones with little or no repair capability. In other instances, obvious rip-offs occur which could be prevented with more stringent oversight by regulatory agencies. Construction and design standards are needed, on the one hand, and consumer reports for disabled people, on the other, if consumer confidence in the products of disability R&D is to be enhanced.

Some Continuing Issues

Aside from stimulation of more and improved research and technology, we need to address some trenchant ethical and technical questions relating to disability concerns. Prominent among these is the economic issue of investing relatively large sums of money in life-saving and adaptive equipment. Another is the extent to which adaptations are to be preferred when such changes come into conflict with the preferences of the larger, nondisabled population.

In an "era of limits," according to some authorities, we must lower our sights and recognize that "we can't solve problems by throwing money at them." Similarly, doctors and medical-ethics specialists are increasingly asking about the wisdom of applying our research-and-technology knowledge to the problem of saving lives at potentially enormous social and economic cost. Rudolf Klein, a professor of social-policy studies at the University of Bath, in the United Kingdom, has proposed that "given the rising cost as well as scope of technology, a policy of striving to prolong every life could cheat others of the opportunity to improve their chances for an active existence." Citing Britain's experience with spina bifida, he notes that a decade ago operations were performed routinely and with great success to save the lives of disabled infants, but that more recently "most physicians here have abandoned the imperative to save every life. Infants with irremediable abnormalities are left untreated, to die usually within nine months or so after birth." Observing that it costs as much as $10,000 annually to maintain a child with spina bifida in an institution, Klein continues: "In my estimation, perhaps the correct conclusion is that Britain, being a relatively poor country, has been compelled to become a pioneer in making the difficult choices in the field of medical care—and that other countries will sooner or later have to follow the example set here."[9]

Similar, albeit less dramatic, questions are being posed with respect to other aspects of disability programming. My own answer revolves around my central belief in the potential of people who are disabled; it is a belief that sustains me in all of my work. And that belief holds that disabled people will achieve to limits defined, not by their disabilities, but by their abilities. To deprive a disabled person of life, or of the education, training, devices, and opportunities he or she needs to maximize those abilities, is to judge him or her not on the basis of what he or she can do, but on the basis of what he or she can't do. An individual with spina bifida has potential, and that potential is what we must develop, nourish, and sustain. For most disabled individuals, the investment will be more than repaid, not only in economic terms through employment and income taxes, but in less tangible human and social returns. A decade ago we thought that most retarded individuals could never be expected to work; today we know that is wrong. Ten years from now, we may know how to prevent and even cure spina bifida, retardation, deafness, and other disabilities. So for all of these reasons, nothing, surely not economic concerns, can deter us from doing what we can to rehabilitate people who are disabled.

A related set of questions arises when the needs of disabled and nondisabled persons appear to clash. Take, for example, the issue of captioning television programs for deaf people. "Open" captioning, such as is used on the

"ABC Evening News" rebroadcast shown on PBS on week-nights, appears on all screens tuned to a particular PBS station or network. While the captions enable people who cannot hear to understand the program, surveys show that a sizable minority (10% to 20% in most cases) of the hearing audience expresses some degree of dissatisfaction with the captions. Some find it "distracting," while others are sufficiently annoyed to switch channels. The question becomes: "Do the benefits accruing to deaf people outweigh the disadvantages or unhappiness for hearing people"? All three commercial television networks answered, in effect, no. They have consistently refused to permit open captions, on the ground that even a 10% dissatisfaction rate would have large implications for advertising revenues and audience-share ratios. The problem is not primarily one of the costs of captioning—$500 per half hour, which is vanishingly small compared to production and other costs associated with television—but of the cost of losing the larger audience. This particular problem, and the way the commercial networks reacted to it, led to further development of "closed" captioning technology, in which only persons who purchase a decoder (or "black box") see the captions. Thus, in this instance, deaf people were required to forego readily available technology, await the uncertain future of a different technology, and, in addition, purchase expensive special devices—all of this despite the fact that the normally hearing population might have become accustomed to, and even benefited from, open captions once they had become more familiar.

The clash appears in other areas as well. The removal of architectural and transportation barriers as required by section 504 of the Rehabilitation Act of 1973, as amended, incurs certain costs, as we will see in the next chapter. Despite the fact, and it is a well documented one, that nondisabled people often enjoy and benefit from barrier-free design, barrier removal will not become widespread in the private as well as the public sector until the general public appreciates its importance to them as well as to disabled people. Acceptance of new technologies will be most rapid when these are designed and marketed with the needs and desires of the larger population at least as firmly in mind as those of the disabled population.

To date, we have not been able to publicize the broad benefits of research, technology, and barrier-removal efforts sufficiently well to help the American people appreciate the urgency of these endeavors. One result may be seen in the President's Fiscal Year 1980 Budget. He proposes spending only $27.5 million on rehabilitation research, down from the 1979 request of $31.5 million, and less even than the amount spent ten years earlier. In fact, because of inflation, the purchasing power of the funds requested is only half that of the 1969 sum. A second result may be seen in the plethora of on-the-shelf technology and devices, prototypes which if mass produced would contribute greatly to the welfare of disabled and elderly Americans, while cutting social-security and other costs considerably. Neither the general public nor private industry has shown much interest in production and distribution of these machines, largely because they do not know their value and because they do not appreciate the true size of the market for these devices.

Research and technology hold great promise of enhancing the lives of disabled and elderly Americans while also helping to eradicate disability itself, both through prevention and through cure. Yet this potential will not be realized until we resolve the ethical questions that continue to plague us, understand better the cost-benefit savings made possible by new technology, communicate the possibilities research offers for disabled and elderly people to the country at large and, through all of these efforts, increase considerably our investment in disability R&D. Few steps would help us so much to add life to years, as we have added years to life.

Meeting the Challenge: Research and Development

I have said that research and development are potentially the most exciting and dramatic steps we can take to help disabled people move from dependence to independence. More precisely, we can invest new resources in prevention and cure, educational techniques, rehabilitation procedures, barrier-removal techniques, and the development, production, and distribution of devices and other equipment. These kinds of research and development activities are at present grossly underfunded.

As part of the ten-year, five-point $22 billion-a-year plan, I suggest we allocate, on the federal, state, local, and private levels, a total of $11 billion in new funding. The investment would rise rapidly until 1987 and then begin to decline as we apply the new techniques, procedures, and devices to reduce other expenditures and as the innovations begin to pay for themselves. Thus, a reading machine developed for blind individuals might be purchased by these persons, schools, rehabilitation agencies, voluntary associations, and other facilities serving blind persons, who in turn will save money they now spend on readers and brailling or recording of written materials.

The decline would not be as steep as in some other areas for two reasons. First, procedures and devices developed on the basic, applied, and prototype research levels during the first several years must be packaged and distributed before the return on investment will begin. Second, research and development historically have generated as many questions as answers. That is, there will be a continuing process of refinement, improvement, and replacement of both ideas and machines throughout the decade. Nevertheless, our investment in research and development may continue to fall in constant dollars, although inflation may force a plateau or rise in actual dollars, because after ten years of activity supported on the levels suggested, we shall have provided to several millions of disabled people opportunities, instruments, and machines enabling them to overcome the effects of their disability and we shall have reduced, substantially, both the prevalence and incidence of disability in our country.

Specifically, I am proposing that we allocate for research, on the federal, state, local, and private levels, $500 million in new spending in 1981, $750 million in 1982, $1 billion in 1983, $1.25 billion in 1984, $1.5 billion in 1985–87, $1.25 billion in 1988, $1 billion in 1989, and $750 million in 1990. All figures are in constant dollars. I have not taken the effect of inflation into account because estimates of the rate of inflation during the 1980s vary widely and wildly. The $11 billion ten-year plan would greatly enhance our ability to rehabilitate disabled and elderly people.

Please note that these are totals for spending on four levels. In the case of research and development, the bulk of the new spending I am proposing will be borne by the federal and private levels, with relatively modest expenditures by state and local governments. The funds are in addition to the amounts now appropriated or projected for 1980. That is, this is new spending.

I anticipate that our investment during the coming decade will quickly become a negative cost. With declines in prevalence and incidence rates; with cuts in social-service and education spending for reading, sign-language interpreting, and attendant care, as equipment to perform many of the tasks these people now do becomes available; with the return from dependence rolls to payrolls of persons who would be enabled to work; and with other factors, we would actually be spending less on research than we would be receiving because of it. The impact may be particularly strong on social-security expenditures, but it will also be felt in other entitlement and discretionary programs.

Support for research and development is but one of the five points of the ten-year plan. It does not help to give a disabled or elderly person an employment-related device if he has not been trained for work; similarly, no amount of research on teaching techniques will be effective if persons who are on dependence rolls have no incentive to leave them and enter educational and rehabilitation programs, or if environmental barriers prevent their doing so.

"The new [section 504] regulations announce the beginning of a costly but welcome era. Nothing the Carter administration will do in the next three years will touch as many lives that are ready for a touch of justice."

George F. Will[1]

3 The Barriers Come Tumbling Down

Of all the complex issues surrounding the problem of disability in our society, none generates such intense emotions or so probing a re-examination of policy as that of barrier removal. Crystallized in its purest form in the debate over access to transportation, because there the conflict in values is sharpest and the financial repercussions most severe, the confrontation between deeply held beliefs occasioned by the barrier-removal provisions of section 504 and other civil-rights statutes offers us perhaps our most finely tuned indicator of the direction we shall take in the 1980s toward people who are disabled.

Paradoxically, the debate is rarely understood even by the protagonists on its front lines, perhaps because the ideas involved are so basic as to stimulate little if any awareness. For section 504 and related laws mandate treatment of disabled people based upon convictions which are at once so central to the founding philosophies of our country as to be accepted without question and yet so diametrically opposed to similarly unquestioned beliefs which have

guided our nation's policies toward disabled people virtually from the beginning as to produce deep dissonance
and moral confusion when brought to consciousness.

Consider for example an incident which occurred during
half-time of a recent Washington Redskins–Kansas City
Chiefs football game in RFK Stadium in Washington, D.C.
As thirty-seven thousand fans watched, two white-coated
attendants helped two young people onto the field. The
band played "You'll Never Walk Alone" as the two young-
sters, one in a wheelchair and the other with crutches,
reached midfield. Both were, a Shriners' announcer told
us, just like the kids our dollars are intended to help. As
the band switched to "The Theme from Rocky," the announcer added: "And this is what your dollars can do!"
The one youngster dropped his crutches, the other rose
from his wheelchair, and together they walked off the
field.

Almost without exception, those in attendance accepted
the Shriners' presentation with sympathy tinged with guilt.
This was, of course, the objective: these are emotions that
translate easily into dollars. The exceptions? Three disabled adults sitting in the bleacher section could barely
suppress their rage at this portrayal of dependent subhu-
man beings magically transformed into "real people" by
the helping hands, and dollars, of able-bodied persons.
It is in this slightly bizarre twist on the Tiny Tim saga
that we can envision the underlying conflict created by
the promulgation of sections 501, 502, 503, and 504 of
the Rehabilitation Act of 1973.[2]

For these statutes require treatment of people who are
disabled not according to the disability and not from the
perspective of the omnipresent helping hand, but with full

equality and access to the mainstream of American society. The central theses of these recent civil-rights enactments are founded in a conviction that separate-but-equal is a patently pernicious premise, an essential contradiction in terms, and an unreachable objective. These statutes proclaim the goal to be one of offering full access to the programs and activities supported by federal funds, and they reject, firmly, the contention that rights may be protected in segregated, separate, and "special" environments. Inherent in these laws is the belief that disabled people are, first of all, people and citizens just as are all others in our society and that, therefore, they must be accorded full participation as equals in the activities made available to others in our country. Stated in this fashion, the foundations of section 504 and the related statutes may appear self-evident on their face, and indeed, in one sense, they are. Yet they are manifestly at odds with the philosophies which have shaped the institutions through which our society treats disabled people. Presented in rather glaring terms in the Shriners' half-time promotion, these beliefs center around the tenet that disabled people are, first of all, disabled individuals who are less to be expected to help themselves than to be accorded special assistance and support until they have become like the rest of us, that is, until they are no longer disabled, and that, therefore, until they have reached that stage, they should be sheltered in some way, protected, and cared for, preferably in settings especially designed to cater to their particular needs. This approach finds one manifestation, when applied to such problems as placement of mentally retarded or mentally ill individuals, in the response "anywhere but here," which in turn produces massive institutions housing these individuals, so that they will not reside "here," in the community.

The two approaches—one stressing the rights of citizens and the other stressing the unique needs of impaired persons—are both firmly rooted in the American experience. Yet it is the latter and not the former that is rooted as well in our history of treatment for people who are disabled. The application of the logical extension of our beliefs in equality before the law to the disabled segment of our society produces strong emotional reactions for precisely this reason. The shift required by the new laws is expressed concisely in the slogan adopted by many disabled individuals: "You gave us your dimes. Now give us our rights." The remnants of the "special" approach, however, make many Americans less generous with their respect than with their dollars. This, too, was exemplified, perhaps more grossly than might be wished, in the Shriners' benefit performance. Few of the observers considered the episode obscene. But the disabled viewers did—as an exploitation reminiscent of "Hey, boy" treatment of blacks.

Interestingly, although these are the fundamental issues at stake with section 504 and related statutes, the debate that is taking place today is not couched in these terms. Rather, it is presented, by both sides, in economic and political arguments. Perhaps this is to be expected in so economically oriented a society as ours. But the debate cannot be understood, or resolved, on this level for the simple reason that it is not here, but on the philosophical bases, that the conflict hinges. This is not to refute the contention that important financial and policy issues are involved; they are, and in many instances these issues are complicated and pervasive in their impact. But it is to say that to resolve these concerns we must address the more fundamental values question. That resolution will determine the direction our nation will pursue and the point of departure it will adopt with respect to the economic and political problems at stake. And because one-quarter of the elderly population is also disabled, the way we resolve those problems will have a powerful effect upon our treatment of old people as well.

Four Statutes

The most important civil-rights provision ever enacted on behalf of disabled people required just one sentence: "No otherwise qualified handicapped individual . . . shall . . . be excluded from participation in, be denied the benefits of, or be subjected to discrimination under any program or activity receiving federal financial assistance." Section 504 was the final sentence of the Rehabilitation Act of 1973 (P.L. 93–112). The following year, while amending the act, Congress held hearings on the statute and made clear its intention that compliance should be forthcoming. Twenty-eight federal agencies are required to promulgate rules applying this sentence to the programs they administer and support.

Two million companies, from small spare-parts manufacturers to huge international corporations, are required to follow equity guidelines in the recruitment, hiring, placement, and advancement of disabled individuals under the terms of section 503. The firms must modify worksites and other facilities to accommodate the special needs of disabled employees, so that they may perform the work for which they were trained. The Department of Labor coordinates the enforcement of all governmental contracts and subcontracts subject to the statute.

More than 450,000 federally owned and leased facilities authorized by 150 programs and operated by 72 agencies must comply with accessibility standards enforced by the Architectural and Transportation Barriers Compliance Board under section 502. The statute is designed to ensure that disabled people, both citizens seeking access to government and federal employees, will enjoy barrier-free entry to the seats of government.

Nondiscrimination in employment is required of every federal department and agency under section 501. The statute is designed to help the federal government become a "model employer" of disabled individuals, setting an example for the private sector.

These four provisions of the Rehabilitation Act form the cornerstone of civil rights for disabled Americans. While there are other critically important rights guaranteed by law, notably those in education mandated by P.L. 94–142 and P.L. 94–482, the four statutes in Title V of the 1973 rehabilitation law are the most central. The four taken together augur the first genuine equality of opportunity America has granted its disabled citizens in more than two hundred years. The rules require the removal of architectural, attitudinal, communication, education, employment, and transportation barriers. They protect disabled people against unjust discrimination and unnecessary obstacles. *If they are followed through in brick and mortar as they are proposed in ink and paper, they will bring about perhaps the greatest civil-rights advance our country has ever known.*

Section 504

Despite the fact that section 504 was enacted in 1973, it was not until almost four years later that the first set of regulations governing its implementation was issued. The Department of Health, Education, and Welfare, under intense pressure from disabled people, released the first rules on April 28, 1977. The following January, the agency issued guidelines for twenty-seven other agencies to follow in drafting similar regulations. These guidelines were based upon Executive Order 11914, issued in 1976 by then-President Gerald Ford, naming HEW "lead agency" on section 504. Among the twenty-seven other agencies required to write section 504 regulations are the Departments of Agriculture, Commerce, Defense, Housing and Urban Development, Justice, Labor, State, Transportation, and the Veterans Administration. P.L. 95–602, the Rehabilitation, Comprehensive Services, and Developmental Disabilities Amendments of 1978, extended the coverage of section 504 to the federal agencies themselves, as well as to their grant recipients.

The HEW guidelines instruct each agency to draft a proposed regulation, hold a public comment period, and, within 135 days of the closing of the comment period, publish final regulations governing how section 504 will be applied to its grant and other fiscal-assistance programs.

All states, counties, cities, public and private agencies, institutions, organizations, firms, or persons to which federal financial assistance is extended directly or through another recipient will be subject to rules developed by the department from which funds are received. The term "federal financial assistance" is defined to mean any grant, loan, contract (other than a procurement contract or contract of insurance or guaranty), or any other arrangement by which an agency provides or otherwise makes available assistance in the form of funds, services of federal personnel, or real and personal property.

The rules issued by the different agencies must be consistent with those of HEW. If the regulations diverge markedly, the result will be chaos for states, cities, and other large entities receiving funds from more than one agency. More serious, the rights of disabled people will be gravely jeopardized. Conversely, uniform and coherent rules will provide readily understood and applied procedures through which recipients may come into compliance, not only with one agency, but with all from whom funds are or may be obtained.

The fact that virtually every major federal agency is required by the executive order, the HEW guidelines, and P.L. 95–602 to develop similar regulations on removing discrimination on the basis of disability provides an unprecedented opportunity for disabled people to secure from the federal government and recipients of federal funds a consistent and readily understood policy for the first time in this country's history. And because virtually every aspect of American life, from transportation to housing, education to employment, health care to veterans programs, is subsidized at least in part by federal funds, this policy will have a massive impact upon the lives of disabled Americans.

Announcing the issuance of the HEW section 504 regulation, Secretary Joseph A Califano, Jr., declared: "The 504 regulation attacks the discrimination, the demeaning practices and the injustices that have afflicted the nation's handicapped citizens. It reflects the recognition of the Congress that most handicapped persons can lead proud and productive lives, despite their disabilities. It will usher in a new era of equality for handicapped individuals in which unfair barriers to self-sufficiency and decent treatment will begin to fall before the force of law."

The HEW regulation established new rights and hastened the enforcement of existing rights in the areas of health services, education, and welfare and other social services. The April 28, 1977, announcement triggered anguished cries from many recipients of grants from the agency, fears that were founded upon the belief that the rules would make huge expenditures necessary. Yet Califano held firm: "Ending discriminatory practices and providing equal access to programs may involve major burdens on some recipients. Those burdens and costs, to be sure, provide no basis for exemption from section 504 or this regulation: Congress' mandate to end discrimination is clear." He estimated that the costs associated with the changes required by the regulation would be approximately $2.4 billion, with most expenses to be incurred by educational facilities.

The regulation not only prohibits discrimination but also requires that disabled people be given the opportunity to participate in programs supported by HEW funds in the most integrated setting possible—and that these services and benefits be as meaningful and effective for disabled persons as they are for other people. "Separate but equal" as a basis for service delivery is expressly banned unless it is required in order for the individual needs of particular disabled persons to be met to the same extent as the needs of others served are met. All new facilities must be barrier free while existing facilities must be adapted so that the programs or activities housed there are accessible to disabled people. Examples of adaptation might be reassignment of classes and, in some cases, home visits. No exceptions to the program accessibility requirement are allowed.

The HEW regulation also mandates equal employment opportunity. The hiring practices set forth are modelled after those established by Title VI of the 1964 Civil Rights Act. These practices were perhaps most graphically described by Chief Justice Warren Burger in *Griggs v. Duke Power Company:*

> Congress has now provided that tests or criteria for employment may not provide equality of opportunity merely in the sense of the fabled offer of milk to the stork and the fox. On the contrary, Congress has now required that the posture and condition of the job-seeker be taken into account. It has—to resort again to the fable—provided that the vessel in which the milk is proffered be one all seekers can use.[3]

In order to ensure equal employment opportunity for disabled people, the HEW regulation prescribes practices in recruitment, advertising, hiring, promotions, transfers, rates of pay, fringe benefits, job definitions, job assignments, vacations, training, and any other terms or conditions of employment that may affect a disabled individual.

All programs and activities subject to the regulation are expected to provide communication accessibility for deaf and blind persons. This may be done through the use of teletypewriters (TTYs) enabling deaf people to use the telephone, sign-language interpreters for classroom use, braille and recordings for blind persons, and other auxiliary aids.

The requirements apply on behalf of "qualified" disabled persons. That is, disabled individuals who have established eligibility for services (they meet all of the usual qualifications and regulations) must receive these services, while those who are qualified for employment must be hired in the same ways as are nondisabled persons. Thus, a deaf person who qualifies for admission into Harvard University has the right to expect the university to provide him with a sign-language interpreter in his classes and other essential educational activities. Similarly, a blind person who is the best qualified candidate for an opening for a social worker in a welfare agency cannot be denied employment on the basis of disability.

Implementation and enforcement of the HEW regulation was slow at first, due in part to the newness of the concepts proposed and in part to the agency's internal difficulties in organizing for the effort. A December 29, 1977, court order by U.S. District Court Judge John Pratt, however, required HEW to eliminate its backlog of cases promptly and to process all new complaints expeditiously. The order took effect almost one year later owing to the fact that 898 additional staff members were required for implementation of the requirements. All complete complaints—those specifying the complainant by name and address, describing or identifying those injured by the alleged discrimination (names are not required), and identifying the institution or individual said to have discriminated, in sufficient detail to inform HEW what discrimination took place and when—must be acknowledged within fifteen days and a determination made as to whether discrimination has in fact occurred within 105 days of receipt of the complaint. Equally important, the court order authorizes HEW to conduct compliance reviews of recipients to assess implementation of the law. This is critical, because complaints usually come from relatively sophisticated persons, while the poorer and less well educated individuals who most frequently are victims of discrimination never complain. If a violation is found to have occurred, HEW will enter into negotiations with the institution and, if compliance has not been secured within 195 days of receipt of the complaint, formal enforcement action will be initiated, including administrative procedures and termination of funds, no later than 225 days after receipt of the original complaint. The court order thus assures disabled people of prompt, appropriate investigation of alleged violations of section 504.

The Pratt decision applies to many other departments and agencies as well because these have agreements with HEW under which enforcement is conducted through HEW's Office for Civil Rights. It is significant, also, because it marks the first time that goals and timetables have been applied to enforcement of a civil-rights statute specifically affecting disabled people. Under Title VI of the 1964 Civil Rights Act, as implemented by HEW, goals and timetables had been applied for many years; women had enjoyed similar protection under Title IX of the Education Amendments. In effect, the fact that goals and timetables were followed for blacks and women, but not for disabled people, created a situation in which investigation of violations of the rights of disabled people took, in practice, lower priority than did those of women and blacks. The Pratt

consent decree, however, effectively terminates this ine-
quality in enforcement and places section 504, Title VI,
and Title IX on an equal footing.

As the twenty-seven other agencies developed, proposed, and then promulgated regulations in compliance
with the executive order, three decisions made by HEW
in the course of developing its own rules and in the drafting
of the guidelines assumed critical importance. The first
was essentially that costs could not be considered to be
a major factor in the protection of the rights of disabled
people. This decision followed recent Supreme Court rul-
ings that money cannot be a reason for the abrogation
of constitutionally guaranteed rights. The agencies could
consider costs, of course, but only costs which would not
have the effect of denying equality of treatment. One result
of the decision is that some agencies have decided to
spread out over a period of years the time allowed for
compliance, in order to help recipients reduce annual outlays. The second key decision was that section 504 applied
to all programs and activities, not only to some. This decision had great impact upon the transportation rules, because it meant that subways as well as buses had to be
made accessible to disabled people. A third HEW decision,
however, limited the scope of section 504's impact: this
was the determination that contracts of insurance or guaranty were not covered. With respect to the Department
of Housing and Urban Development's regulation, this decision meant that the bulk of the department's financial support of housing, that of federally insured loans, would not
be covered, and therefore the only housing subject to section 504 would be that constructed or modified with federal
grants.

Controversy over 504

Section 504 has generated considerable press coverage, both for its important provisions protecting disabled people from unjust discrimination and for the problems associated to date with its implementation.[4] All major court cases involving section 504 have upheld its central tenets and those of the agency regulations. Yet the issue remains "hot copy" because of the huge price tags alleged to be involved and the disruptions that may be caused by its implementation. The controversies may be illustrated by consideration of two instances, one concerning retarded individuals and the other relating to transportation of physically disabled persons.

On December 23, 1977, U.S. District Court Judge James Broderick ruled that section 504 of the Rehabilitation Act prohibits segregation of services for retarded persons at Pennhurst Center, Spring City, Pennsylvania. Basing his decision upon what Justice Department attorney Arthur Peabody called "the most complete record of any right-to-treatment case tried in the United States in any Federal District Court," Judge Broderick established with his opinion a powerful precedent which potentially affects every institution in the United States that serves retarded individuals—and many that serve other disabled persons. Eighty witnesses, including fourteen international experts, testified in the nine-week trial.

The case was the first in which a federal district court considered the legislative history and the HEW regulation on section 504, the first to apply the statute to a large class of disabled individuals, and the first to establish that section 504 orders community-based, small-scale, and integrated services to all retarded individuals on an equal basis.

Testimony revealed that costs are almost halved when retarded persons reside in and are served by the community as opposed to being institutionalized in Pennhurst. More important, the individuals are likely to attain a higher level of functioning and of independence when mainstreamed than when institutionalized. By contrast, treatment in a massive and segregated setting often produces actual deterioration in social skills and other competencies. Clearly, community-based programs benefit both retarded persons and society at large.

The Broderick opinion is particularly significant because Pennsylvania, according to the President's Committee on Mental Retardation, is one of the nation's best states in provision of quality care in institutions. Thus, if Pennhurst violates section 504, the 180 other institutions throughout the country which serve more than 238,000 individuals are also likely in violation.

State and local defendants were unable to produce even a single witness who would refute the plaintiffs' charges. Said Pennhurst superintendent Duane Youngberg: "I don't think there should be a Pennhurst. In a large, residential facility, good care is an almost impossible task. Theoretically, all of these people should be living in the community." Added the Pennsylvania deputy attorney general representing the state defendants: "The Commonwealth is quite simply not defending Pennhurst."[5]

Despite all of this, community reaction to the decision impelled Pennsylvania to appeal the decision. The reaction raises intriguing questions about how the Broderick decision, if it is upheld, will be implemented. If institutionalization without regard for provision of equal services violates section 504 and other prohibitions against segregation on the basis of disability, what kinds of community-based programs would be in compliance with the law—and acceptable enough to community residents to have a chance for success? Mainstreaming of retarded adults in an America frequently hostile to such integration appears more likely to succeed in towns like Waterbury, Vermont, where residents have had since 1891 to become accustomed to seeing retarded persons in their neighborhoods because of the presence of the Vermont State Hospital, than in places like Suffolk County, Long Island, where state efforts to rent a private home as a hostel for nine retarded adults produced strong community objections. And the problem of providing supportive services that are of high quality and ready availability in cities and towns across the nation has yet to be solved satisfactorily.

If the Pennhurst case illustrated the fact that costs alone are not an overriding concern of the American people (it is much less expensive to mainstream than to institutionalize, yet mainstreaming is unacceptable to many persons), transportation of physically disabled persons offers an example of a controversy in which the costs are almost the only aspect of section 504 that is being debated. Still, the fear instilled by mainstreaming is a hidden agenda item assuming major but largely unrecognized importance in the discussion.

Two issues have dominated the debate on transportation. One has to do with bus design and centers upon the "Transbus," a bus designed at a cost of $27 million over eight years by the Department of Transportation (DOT). The second, in which Transbus plays a large part, is the department's section 504 regulation. The costs associated with this regulation are estimated variously at $2 billion to $8 billion depending upon who is doing the estimating (the lower estimate is that of the department; the higher that of the public-transit authorities).

Transbus, the result of five separate congressional mandates, is the first fully accessible standard-size bus to be designed in this country. It offers passengers a ride approaching in quality that of private automobiles, while reducing trip time and other transit costs. While the initial purchase price is somewhat higher than currently available buses ($120,000 v. $100,000), the lower operating, repair, and other costs together with increased ridership (estimated at 10% over current figures, in addition to the disabled and elderly riders newly attracted by the accessibility provisions) will more than make up for the higher capital investment. The wide doors, low floors, and front-door ramps for accessibility enable as many as 13.3 million persons not now able to take full advantage of urban mass transportation to ride the bus. Because 80% of all people using public transportation use buses, the potential impact upon disabled people, enabling them to get to and from educational, employment, and cultural programs and facilities, is enormous.

Transbus, then, seems to have it all. It enables virtually everyone to use the bus, thus appealing powerfully to our sense of equality of opportunity. For nondisabled persons, it provides faster, more comfortable, and safer rides than are now available. For disabled people, it offers truly accessible public transportation that was never before possible. And the cost-benefit ratios are unassailable, because the bus is less expensive over time than currently marketed vehicles.

Yet the bus stirred massive, prolonged opposition from

two segments of American society: the urban mass-transportation authorities and General Motors. The transit officials, led by their association, the American Public Transit Association (APTA), waged fierce war against Transbus over a period of several years. The opposition appeared to be centered upon a contention that the bus was both too expensive and unworkable as a solution to the transit needs of disabled people. B. R. Stokes, the association's executive vice-president, argued that the very idea of federal requirements in bus design was erroneous: that Washington could "mandate a panacea" was "absolute nonsense," he said. "The imposition of any program which would imply the use of scarce federal resources, for what we believe is a non-solution in the first place, borders on the ridiculous," he added, directing his comments as much to DOT's section 504 rules as to Transbus itself. What was APTA's solution? The association stressed "dial-a-ride" small-van programs and related segregated services as an alternative and pressed for what it called "local option" in deciding how to meet the transportation needs of disabled people.

General Motors' opposition was no less heated. Aiming its charges both at DOT and the Congress, GM blasted the Transbus design and proposed its own in its stead. The GM bus, "RTS II," would have a lift, not a ramp, and the lift was to be installed in the rear door, not the front door, of the bus. During the summer of 1978, GM succeeded in convincing the Congress to introduce an amendment to the Surface Mass Transportation Amendments which would require DOT to "reevaluate" the Transbus mandate. Congressional investigation of the charges proved that GM's version would unnecessarily disrupt bus service by requiring the bus driver to stop the bus, lock the front door and the fare box, walk to the back of the bus, operate the mechanism, help the person board, return the lift mechanism to the original position, walk back to the front of the bus and unlock the front door and the fare box, all of which would take three to five minutes. Transbus's ramp, by contrast, offers disabled people entry and exit in a matter of five seconds. The time, labor, and service interruption considerations led the Congress to drop GM's amendment and to support DOT's original mandate.[6]

The Transbus debate illustrates in an interesting way how costs and other surface considerations may obscure deeper, more emotional issues. After meeting with representatives of disabled people, both APTA and GM eventually conceded that the arguments they had been using were without sufficient validity. What, then, gave rise to them in the first place? The APTA solution, that of separate "dial-a-ride" services, takes disabled people out of the mainstream system. This is a critical point: bus operators who feel uncomfortable with the prospect of disabled persons boarding their vehicles, and bus owners who fear loss of general riders if disabled persons were to begin using the mass-transit buses, may have had separation in mind from the beginning. And it cannot be totally a coincidence that GM's lift mechanism was placed not in the front, but in the rear, of the bus. The parallel to the Freedom Rides of the sixties is obvious.

Similar concerns permeate the debate on DOT's section 504 regulation. The huge price tags, if accurate, would provide such a powerful argument that the philosophical and moral bases may be obscured. New York City Mayor

Ed Koch told DOT that implementing the rules as proposed would cost as much as $2 billion in New York City alone. "Such a burden would literally bankrupt us," he testified. The Chicago Transit Authority claimed that retrofitting its rapid-rail system would cost $910 million and pointedly remarked that this sum exceeded the total invested in the system since 1890. APTA, adding up the claims from the different transit authorities, testified that the rules would cost as much as $8 billion to implement. Columnist Neal Pierce, writing in the Washington *Post* and other newspapers, called upon the government to "cease and desist" with the DOT section 504 rules: "President Carter has a golden opportunity to show his mettle on fighting inflation, reducing burdensome regulation, saving energy and helping out the nation's cities. But he'll have to pay a price: offending the wheelchair lobby."[7]

The huge cost estimates derive principally from figures based upon the expenditures needed to retrofit subways in five cities which have old, inaccessible systems. In fact, 90% of the estimated cost associated with the DOT rules are funds that would be needed for subway retrofit. The APTA and transit authority estimates are exaggerated because they include renovation costs that would be assumed in any event, even if section 504 were not in effect, and ignore the fact that designing for access costs no more than designing inaccessible facilities. The retrofit costs are overblown as well, as the rules require this only when no other way can be found to make the system accessible and when renovation occurs. Considerable time is allowed by the rules, thus permitting the authorities to spread out the work. Finally, DOT pays 80% of the capital costs, with the cities and states splitting the remaining portion. Despite all of this, the amount of money needed is not the

central issue, however large the dollar figures are. This
is what so few people understand. The key point is that
tax dollars paid by American citizens are used to construct
and operate subway as well as other mass transportation
facilities and vehicles; what the Congress has said is that
tax dollars cannot be spent to benefit only some of the
people who need assistance, but must be allocated in such
a way that all citizens can benefit. Thus, even if the time
period is extended over several decades, the only legal
approach is to make the system accessible.

The irony is that, looking at the overall picture, it is
economically more prudent to mainstream disabled people
into the general transportation system than it is to segre-
gate them. Startling as the mainstreaming costs may be,
they are minuscule compared with segregation costs. Consider, for example, the costs of APTA's "dial-a-ride" option. By the association's own estimate (which is almost
certain to be conservative), dial-a-ride would cost $1.75
billion per year. Thus, in ten years, it would cost six times
as much as would mainstreaming; in twenty years, almost
thirteen times as much. Designing for access involves one-
time costs for renovation and design; thereafter, no appreciable additional expenses are involved. Special services,
by contrast, require extra vehicles, more manpower, additional fuel, and other operating and maintenance costs,
and these costs are continuing, year-after-year, expenses.
Interestingly, APTA may be cutting the operators' throats
by pushing this option because of the peculiarities of federal financing of transportation. Whereas DOT pays 80%
of capital costs for construction and renovation, the bulk
of what is needed for mainstreaming, this is not true of
the annual costs of dial-a-ride services, which must be
borne almost entirely by the local transit authorities.

APTA's hope apparently is that if their option is approved, the funding rules will be changed, but the gamble serves to illustrate the lengths to which the association and its members are willing to go to avoid mainstreaming disabled people into the general system. This exemplifies, again, the fundamental nature of the philosophical and moral issues raised by section 504.

The ways in which our society resolves issues such as those posed by Pennhurst and DOT's regulation will indicate strongly how it will handle other aspects of the problem of disability. For the possible future emerges in vivid detail in the *Federal Register*'s narrow columns announcing the 504 regulations, the glittering goals almost obscured in the painstaking precision of hundreds of pages of fine print and cost-benefit analyses. There are rules on telephones and teletypewriters, rest rooms and restaurants, schools and subways, hospitals and hostels, bus terminals and airline terminals. There are regulations on education and employment, recreation and leisure, agriculture and commerce, housing and transportation, defense and veterans affairs. And these rules apply to all federal agencies which give grants, as well as to states, counties, cities, institutions, public and private agencies, organizations, firms, and persons receiving them. Whether these rules are followed, whether the proposed procedures are implemented, then, will reveal a great deal about how ready we are to extend "a touch of justice" to disabled Americans.

Section 503

Every employer doing business with the federal government under a contract exceeding $2,500 is required to take "affirmative action" to hire disabled people, promote disabled employees, and provide placement, advanced training, and other opportunities to disabled workers on the same basis as is done for other workers. The section 503 provisions of the Rehabilitation Act of 1973, as amended, have been much less controversial than have those under section 504. Nevertheless, major problems have surfaced which must be addressed immediately.

The Department of Labor's Office of Federal Contract Compliance Programs (OFCCP), which administers section 503, conducted a pilot survey in 1978 of three hundred large, medium, and small contractors and subcontractors. While the sample was too restricted to permit confident projections to be made on the basis of the results, the findings are still important. More than 90% of all firms surveyed were not in full compliance with the 1973 statute and the 1974 regulations. At about the same time, a second major problem emerged: surprisingly few disabled people were identifying themselves as disabled in order to claim protection under the statute. Their reluctance appears to reflect their doubt that the firms would protect their rights and that the Department of Labor would enforce the law. These two problems continue to plague implementation of section 503.

Fortunately, the department has taken vigorous steps to do what it could to ensure more rapid and uniform implementation. A series of seventeen thousand directed compliance reviews, in which firms selected at random are visited on site by compliance officers, has been inaugurated. An intensive training program has begun to familiarize OFCCP personnel with the law and the regulations. A new set of revised rules has been promulgated which strengthens some of the more glaring weaknesses in the program. And the department has stepped up its technical assistance efforts to train contractors in the law's requirements. Similarly, it has recognized the problem among disabled persons who qualify for, but do not claim, protection and has moved to help to resolve this issue as well. The leadership of some of the nation's largest companies in designing and carrying out innovative hire-the-handicapped programs is beginning to have a powerful effect upon industry generally and provides perhaps the most encouraging evidence that, after more than six years of haphazard and laggard implementation, section 503 may at last begin to stimulate genuine gains in employment among disabled people. Each of these steps will be examined in turn.

Violations. The section 503 regulations require that all phases of employment practices, including hiring, upgrading, transfer, demotion, recruitment, layoff, and termination be covered. In actual practice, many contractors have taken steps in only a few of these areas. A similar problem has emerged with respect to the requirement to examine all recruitment and hiring practices to ensure that all requirements are clearly job related. Many firms have not reviewed their employment procedures, preferring to examine individual jobs subsequent to application by a disabled person for that particular position. The outreach provisions of the law, including use of all possible recruitment sources, is another area in which many contractors fall short; too many continue to look only to their regular sources of applicants, typically state employment agencies and vocational rehabilitation agencies, while neglecting organizations of and for disabled people, publications reaching disabled individuals, and other possible sources of applicants.

One of the most common violations relates to the issue of "reasonable accommodation." The original regulations required that contractors accommodate the mental or physical limitations of disabled persons unless it could be shown that such accommodations would impose an "undue hardship" upon the contractor, that is, if the cost or other requirements would clearly be excessive or impossible to meet. The rules did not, however, explicitly require contractors to make their work facilities accessible to and usable by disabled persons. Thus, many disabled persons were denied employment because they could not even get to the personnel office, not to mention the actual jobsite. The lack of an accessibility standard was a major shortcoming of the original regulation. The just-issued new rules correct this oversight by requiring that certain portions of the facilities, notably the personnel or employment office and some segment of the actual worksite, be made accessible. All new facilities are required to meet minimal accessibility standards. These rules were written in this way because retrofitting existing buildings can be expensive, hence some limitation is needed in the amount of modifications required, whereas designing new facilities for full accessibility costs virtually no more than does planning inaccessible buildings.

Another aspect of the problem with reasonable accommodations is that the original rule offered examples of what this term might mean but nowhere provided an actual definition for it. In fact, the most controversial sections of the original regulation are the least thoroughly explained, while less burdensome requirements are spelled out in exhaustive detail. The department should not have been surprised, then, to discover that reasonable accommodation violations were widespread. The new regulation considerably strengthens this area and offers explicit descriptions of what the contractors are expected to do.

Enforcement. From 1974 to 1977, the department relied almost exclusively upon investigation of complaints filed by individuals who believed they had been discriminated against. Virtually no other enforcement tool was being employed. Accordingly, systemic discrimination could not be detected, and only more sophisticated persons, those with the knowledge and political savvy to file complaints, were protected. Clearly neither result was intended by the Congress. When the Carter administration came into office, one of its first steps was to institute a program of directed-compliance reviews, beginning with the three-hundred-firm pilot study and continuing with a much larger annual program.

Similarly, before 1978 virtually no firm was subjected to the statute's penalty—cancellation of the contract and possibly debarment from doing business with the government in the future. The department has now advised firms that cancellations and debarments may occur if and when violations are discovered either through the complaint process or through directed-compliance reviews. The need for such enforcement is clear. Through 1977, only 4,400 complaints were filed in the section 503 program. With more than two million contractors and subcontractors holding in excess of $3 billion worth of contracts potentially affecting as many as four million disabled applicants and employees, the program demonstrably was not reaching its goals. Conducting seventeen thousand reviews annually offers the opportunity that each of the 250,000 major firms covered by section 503 will have its program investigated as often as once every five years. The results should become apparent shortly, particularly if the department follows up on its statement that, should serious violations be found, contracts may be terminated.

Training. As astonishing as it may appear, the department did not begin any serious training of its compliance officers in the statute and regulation implementing section 503 until 1979, instructing only the fifty "specialists" who were responsible for all investigations nationwide. Generalists investigating complaints literally had to read the rules themselves and often were no more able to interpret them properly than were the contractors they were reviewing. Early in 1979, a training manual was developed and federal and regional personnel were provided with in-depth instruction on what to look for and what to do if they found apparent violations. Training for contractors is at least as important: it makes eminently good sense to prevent, rather than just seek to correct, misinterpretations. In 1978 and 1979, the department had accelerated its efforts to ensure that small as well as large firms are provided with solid training in the requirements of the statute. Training for disabled people, another key component of the triangle, has yet to be conducted on anything resembling the scale that will be needed, however, and remains perhaps the most pressing concern, particularly in light of the relative paucity of complaints.

New Rules. The revised section 503 regulations not only correct some of the earlier oversights, notably in accessibility and reasonable accommodation, but also address what was in 1977 and 1978 a serious issue among contractors who also held grants subject to section 504. The two sets of regulations, from two separate departments (the Department of Labor is also issuing a section 504 regulation to cover its grant awards), contained several important differences. The most notable, perhaps, was that section 504, but not section 503, explicitly spelled out what accessibility and reasonable accommodation were to mean. Another area of difference concerned "pre-employment inquiries." Section 503 allowed, while section 504 prohibited, employers asking disabled applicants about the nature of (or existence of) their disability. The new rules offer more congruence between the two sets of requirements.

Private Efforts. Some large companies, notably International Business Machines (IBM) and American Telephone & Telegraph Company (AT&T), had begun intensive hire-the-handicapped programs long before the section 503 regulations became effective. One of the most admirable of these early efforts was that developed by the Chesapeake and Potomac (C&P) Telephone Company in metropolitan Washington, D.C. Its "Handicap Awareness Program" covered all aspects of the hiring process and offered innovative solutions to difficult problems. The program is now being used as a model for many other employers. The importance of these efforts is perhaps most clearly seen in the fact that they represent a genuine, good-faith, and voluntary attempt by a company to employ disabled people at all levels. When more employers hire disabled persons not because they are required to do so by the federal government, but because they believe that it is "good business," we will see remarkable advances in the levels of employment among the disabled population.

Such advances are long overdue. The 1970 census found

that only 42% of the disabled population was even in the labor force, most having given up looking for employment altogether. Such enforced dependency is costing our country hundreds of billions of dollars annually, money we just cannot afford. By contrast, private employment of such persons makes tax-users into tax-payers, reversing the flow of dollars (to the federal treasury in income taxes rather than from the treasury in entitlement benefits), takes people off Medicare and Medicaid programs and places them on private group-health-insurance plans, and at the same time enables other members of the disabled person's family to work rather than having to remain home to care for the dependent individual. The results could be felt by each of us in several hundreds of dollars in reductions in social-security and income taxes if anything like the potential for private employment of disabled people were to be reached.

CONTROVERSY OVER 503

Section 503 has not generated anything approximating the intense and volatile debate that has arisen over section 504. Nevertheless, some salient issues remain unsettled. Perhaps the most serious, as in section 504, relates to costs. Another important concern has to do with insurance coverage and how this affects employment of disabled people.

With respect to costs, all major studies which have been done have revealed that cost estimates anticipated when the law was enacted were greatly overblown. A 1969 Civil Service Commission study of severely disabled federal employees, which found that the actual costs of meeting the accommodation needs of such persons in agency employment were quite low, has proven to apply as well to the private sector. The 1969 survey found that 95% of the employees required neither extensive accessibility nor accommodation to their jobsites, while 3¾% needed accessibility changes only and 1¼% required jobsite accommodations. A National League of Cities study found that it costs less than one-half of one percent of the total cost of constructing a new building to make it completely accessible to and usable by disabled people. Mainstream, Inc., a Washington, D.C., consulting firm, estimates that it costs about 1¢ per square foot per month to make most existing facilities accessible, compared to a monthly cost of 12–13¢ per square foot just to polish floors and clean carpets. The new Department of Labor section 503 regulations insist upon full access in new buildings, recognizing that design for access does not cost appreciably more than does inaccessible design, but permits employers to retrofit only selected areas of existing buildings. Clearly, in view of the costs, these are reasonable requirements.

The insurance issue is more complex. Some firms have complained that if they were to employ severely disabled persons their insurance rates would increase. In some cases this might happen. However, several factors must be kept in mind. First, group insurance, which is typically the form of coverage obtained by private employers, is based upon the record for safety and claims of the entire covered group of workers. Thus, hiring several disabled persons in a work force of several hundreds or thousands will have little effect upon the group rate. Moreover, many insurance carriers encourage employment of disabled people, rather than discourage it. The only notable exceptions relate to persons with terminal illnesses or disabilities expected to result in very heavy medical expenses in the near future. Most disabled persons, particularly those who seek full-time employment, are not likely to require more medical attention than are able-bodied workers. The Department of Labor, like the Department of Health, Education, and Welfare, accordingly requires that contractors or grant recipients whose insurance companies decline to provide coverage for disabled employees must find another carrier who will supply such protection. Insurance issues cannot, by themselves, provide legal justification for refusal to employ a disabled person. Despite all this, the policies of both departments with regard to insurance are constantly under review, and modifications may be made, should insurance practices demand such changes.

The Tax Reform Act of 1976 and other laws offer several possible incentives to employment of disabled persons which address the cost and insurance issues. Landlords and employers may claim as much as $25,000 annually in tax deductions for accessibility modifications through calendar-year 1979. (At the time of this writing, it was not certain whether this provision would be continued for future years.) Similarly, current tax codes offer employers up to $100,000 deductions for salary and fringe benefits incurred in employment of previously unemployed disabled individuals. Because insurance is usually offered as part of a fringe-benefit package, the law helps to resolve this problem as well. Finally, the Rehabilitation, Comprehensive Services, and Developmental Disabilities Amendments of 1978, P.L. 95–602, enact a community employment program for disabled persons in which employers may be reimbursed for the costs they incur in employing disabled persons and any attendants or assistants these workers may require (such as interpreters for deaf persons, readers for blind individuals, and personal-care attendants for people with mobility impairments); the law also offers severely disabled persons who are currently on Medicaid or Medicare the option of continuing to receive these benefits despite the fact that they are working. While restricted in size, the new community employment program will provide us with some answers with respect to the cost effectiveness of these kinds of government assistance designed to stimulate employment of disabled people.

SECTION 502

Sections 502 and 501 differ from sections 504 and 503 in that they deal primarily not with the private sector but with the public sector. That is, section 502 speaks to the issue of accessibility to buildings owned and used by federal agencies, while section 501 relates to federal employment of disabled persons. One would expect that, were the federal government entirely serious about Title V, special emphasis would be placed upon sections 502 and 501, because government cannot realistically expect private employers to follow rules it is not willing itself to observe. Instead, progress on these two statutes has lagged behind that on the other two provisions. This state of affairs cannot continue for much longer without provoking a private-sector revolt against sections 504 and 503.

Section 502 of the Rehabilitation Act of 1973 established an Architectural and Transportation Barriers Compliance Board which was authorized to enforce the Architectural Barriers Act of 1968, a law requiring that federal buildings and facilities be accessible to disabled people. The board began operating in March 1975. It has the power to order accessibility, issue citations of violation of the law, and withhold government funds if necessary to ensure that accessibility is effected.

Problems began almost immediately. The board was given no line-item budget of its own, but instead was forced to compete for support within the U.S. Department of Health, Education, and Welfare appropriations process. Second, the board was composed of representatives of the very federal agencies it was constituted to monitor. Third, these representatives were not given standard-making powers; rather, each agency reserved the right to set its own standards for accessibility. Thus, the board was expected to enforce the 1968 law against its own members, without authority to set the rules under which the enforcement was to take place. As a result, progress for three and a half years was minimal, with agency representatives reluctant to permit their own agencies to be compelled to comply with the law.

Many of these problems were resolved with enactment of the Rehabilitation, Comprehensive Services, and Developmental Disabilities Amendments of 1978 (P.L. 95–602). The membership of the board was expanded to include, in addition to representatives from ten federal agencies, eleven new members drawn from the general public, five of whom are themselves disabled individuals. Thus, a majority of the voting members of the board now are nongovernmental employees who represent the people being affected by and using the buildings and facilities covered by the law. This is expected to assist in the resolution of the conflict-of-interest problem plaguing the board in the past and permit it to move more aggressively against federal agencies alleged to have violated the law.

The board was also authorized to establish minimum standards and guidelines for implementation and enforcement of the 1968 act. Its scope of control was expanded to include not just architectural barriers, but also obstacles confronting deaf and blind individuals ("communication barriers") and transportation barriers. Its budget has also been increased somewhat, although far less than would be required for vigorous enforcement activity.

There is reason to believe, then, that the board will move beyond public-relations gestures and isolated citations to a more concentrated monitoring posture. The urgent need for such aggressiveness is readily apparent when one considers the fact that disabled people, like other citizens, must be able to visit the seats of government in order to transact their business with it, must be able to enter and use federal buildings in order to be able to work as federal employees (a right protected by section 501), and must be able to communicate with their representatives in government. All three areas are severely restricted at present.

Section 501

Disabled people wishing to work in, or secure promotions from, federal agencies are protected under section 501 of the Rehabilitation Act of 1973. The guarantee of nondiscrimination contained there, however, has never been enforced. For more than five years, the government merely asked different agencies to compile annual statistics on the numbers of disabled persons employed that year; many agencies did not even file this voluntary report, while those that did typically reported levels of employment by disabled people hovering around one percent. It was not until March 1978 that the general complaint procedure available to other federal employees was extended to include disabled workers. Clearly, the government has an abysmal record of hiring disabled persons, a record that threatens to destroy its credibility when it insists that private employers subject to sections 503 and 504 employ disabled people. And, while such private organizations and companies are required to accommodate for the impairments of disabled people, making it possible for them to perform jobs for which they are qualified, the federal government itself until 1979 did not even permit employment of sign-language interpreters specifically to translate for deaf workers, readers to work for blind persons, or other basic accommodations and modifications.

Fortunately, legislation enacted in 1978 and implemented in 1979 promises to alter this state of affairs considerably. Many of these improvements were contained in the Rehabilitation, Comprehensive Services, and Developmental Disabilities Amendments of 1978. Section 505(a) (1) of this law extends the remedies, procedures, and rights available to minority-group members and women to protect any disabled applicant or employee of a federal agency who files a complaint of discrimination under section 501. It is now possible for a disabled person to go to court if he is not satisfied with the action taken to resolve his complaint. If the court finds that discrimination has occurred, it may order affirmative action relief including reinstatement or hiring of the complainant. Back pay is provided if applicable; this important provision was never before available to disabled persons under section 501.

Another extremely important advance is contained in

section 505(b). For the first time, a court may allow the prevailing party, other than the federal government, an award of attorney's fees in any action related to Title V of the Rehabilitation Act. One of the greatest problems disabled people who believe they have been victims of discrimination have faced has been that of "inaccessible counsel." That is, lawyers willing to argue their cases have been few and far between. Now that attorney's fees are available, we can expect that disabled complainants will obtain a much more favorable reception when they seek lawyers to assist them in bringing complaints.

The Civil Service Reform Act of 1978 (P.L. 95–454) provides, in section 302, that federal agencies may employ interpreters and readers for deaf and blind persons, or assign such responsibility to already-employed workers as part of their jobs. This provision eliminates the frequently invoked excuse of agencies for not employing communication-limited individuals: that they do not have the legal authority to provide readers or interpreters. Disabled people hired under Schedule A (excepted appointments) may now convert to regular civil-service status after a successful two-year period of employment. This important provision may enable many disabled people who now do not qualify for the same benefits and protection available to other employees to demonstrate that they are qualified for permanent, not just provisional, career civil-service status.

Two other new laws, the Federal Employees' Flexible and Compressed Work Schedules Act of 1978 and the Federal Employees' Part-time Career Employment Act of 1978, will serve to encourage disabled people to seek federal employment by permitting "flextime" work arrangements where needed to allow for transportation to and from work and part-time employment for those not willing or able to work full time.

President Carter's Reorganization Plans Number 1 and Number 2 shift responsibility for section 501 from the Civil Service Commission to the Equal Employment Opportunities Commission and replace the Civil Service Commission with three separate agencies. A Merit System Protection Board will handle all grievances not based solely on discrimination, the Office of Personnel Management will offer technical assistance to and help in management decisions related to section 501 and other matters, and a Federal Labor Relations Authority will handle labor-management issues in federal agencies.

Needed now are steps to translate these new legislative initiatives and reorganization plans into actual procedures protecting the rights of disabled applicants and employees. The next step is to move beyond just nondiscrimination and mandate affirmative action on behalf of disabled people. Only when the federal government expects the same steps from itself—and meets these requirements—can it expect the private sector to take seriously the mandates of sections 503 and 504. As one private employer put it recently: "If the Feds, who are in the business of spending money, can't see the value of hiring disabled people, how can it expect us, who are in the business of making money, to do so?"

Some Next Steps

There exists at this time no federal requirement that private companies not subject to section 503 hire disabled people or make accessibility modifications. Excluded from current law are hundreds of thousands of restaurants, theatres, recreation facilities and parks, private housing units, stores, and small businesses. Yet, it is precisely here that the necessities of "living" as opposed to just "existing," and the amenities that make life enjoyable, fall. Clearly, addition of disability rights to the areas protected under Title VII of the 1964 Civil Rights Act is essential.

Information on barrier-removal needs and techniques remains far behind the demand. Too few architects and engineers know how to design barrier-free environments. Too few builders, buyers, and renters understand the importance, to them, to their families, and to the community, of designing for access to all Americans. Too few administrators and planners know where to go to find information on inexpensive and effective ways to retrofit existing facilities for accessibility. And too few disabled and elderly people are aware of their legal rights of access to government, private companies, and publicly supported programs and activities. For all of these reasons, we need to upgrade considerably our information-and-referral programs on accessibility.

Barrier removal is perhaps the most basic of the needs facing disabled and elderly people today. The flagrant lack of access of most of America produces enormous frustration to persons wanting to get an appropriate education, specific job training, employment commensurate with their abilities, a place to live, transportation to and from work and other facilities, and to live a full and satisfying life in the community.

Yet barrier removal is important for other reasons as well. There are in our country millions of citizens, one out of every nine of us, who are now over the age of sixty-five and who can expect to live for another sixteen years on the average. The number is increasing each year, as the "bubble" produced by the post-World War II baby boom moves across the generations to become a senior boom. Increasing numbers of these elderly citizens are forced into dependence or placed in nursing homes, hospitals, and other institutional settings, not because they are no longer able to function independently, but because they cannot get around our inaccessible communities. With costs for such placement running at levels in excess of $10,000 annually for each person, we must ask whether we can continue to afford these barriers in our homes, cities, and rural areas.

The debate over barriers is turning on costs, but I believe we are looking at the wrong costs. The highest figures I have seen for barrier-removal efforts do not exceed $20 billion over the next decade, or an average of $2 billion annually. *No one has ever said that making America accessible could cost as much as does our inaccessibility now.* My best estimate is that lack of access now costs America more than $100 billion each and every year, with the costs rising to as much as $200 billion a year within the next decade. Thus, the figure with which we must compare the maximum $20-billion figure for a ten-year program of barrier removal is governmental and private spending and lost wages exceeding one thousand billion dollars, or more than $1 trillion. This mind-boggling figure is what we shall spend if we "do nothing"—that is, if we do not remove barriers, bring disabled and elderly people out of segregation and into integration, and help them move from dependence to independence as self-sufficient, taxpaying citizens.

The question is not: Can we afford to make America accessible? Rather it must be: Can we afford not to?

Meeting the Challenge:
Barrier Removal

Eliminating existing architectural, transportation, and communication barriers can be expensive. Combined with other steps proposed in this book, however, the expense will be recovered by society at large. One of the problems in this area is that the people spending the money for barrier removal are not always the same people who benefit financially from this activity. Thus, while a college or university may find its costs repaid in tuition payments received from persons who otherwise would not be able to attend the institution, this might not always be true, and in any event, the repayment would be spread over a period of years. To take another, better, example, a city government that removes barriers in its streets and buildings might not recover the costs. In both cases, there are ways the expenses may be repaid, but in both cases other forces, notably rising energy costs and inflation, have combined to discourage such spending. The explicit requirement of section 504 is that these barriers be removed, and the very important civil-rights prohibition is that these steps not be delayed or foregone merely because of costs. (To permit this would establish a "no pay, no rights" situation in which schools, cities, and others subject to section 504 might continue to violate the rights of disabled people until they receive outside funding for barrier removal.) Nonetheless progress in barrier removal has been slow. How can we break the impasse?

One way might be by extending for another ten years the existing tax deduction permitted landlords who eliminate barriers and increasing the allowable deduction to $50,000 annually. At present, under the Tax Reform Act of 1976, deductions may be taken up to a maximum of $25,000. The provision has been very poorly publicized, so few landlords have learned of its existence, and at any rate it was scheduled for expiration on December 31, 1979. Continuing it and raising the deduction makes sense because barrier removal is in the interest of the United States government, which stands to save many billions of dollars in dependence expenditures. No other segment of American society will benefit quite so greatly; another way of looking at this is to understand that savings by the federal government may produce tax cuts for all of us, both in income taxes and social security taxes. State and local governments may also offer tax deductions for the same reasons, particularly because welfare expenses are largely state and local rather than federal in nature, and barrier removal helps disabled people get off welfare.

I have followed the section 504 timetables rather generally in estimating costs of barrier removal over ten years. I expect that it will cost, on the federal, state, local, and private levels, approximately $14.8 billion over the coming decade to remove most of the more significant barriers preventing disabled people from gaining full access to the community and to employment, educational, medical, and other facilities. Section 504 provides that architectural barriers must be removed within three (in some agencies, more) years when these barriers prevent disabled people from entering into and using the program. Experience indicates that many recipients wait almost the full period allowed them before making these changes. A second factor I have used in calculating these costs is that it will take time for restaurants, theatres, sports facilities, stores, and other facilities and programs to learn of and take advantage of accessibility provisions. Time is also required to assess the need and to design renovations to meet it. Thus, I have proposed that barrier-removal spending increase until about 1984, by which time many of the barriers will have been removed. By 1990, few major barriers should remain.

Specifically, I feel we will need to spend $500 million in 1981, $1 billion in 1982, $2 billion in 1983, $3 billion in 1984, $2 billion in 1985, $1.8 billion in 1986, $1.5 billion in 1987, $1.25 billion in 1988, $1 billion in 1989, and $750 million in 1990 for the barrier-removal phase of the ten-year plan outlined in Chapter 1.

The bulk of these costs will be incurred by small businesses and stores in the community, simply because there are so many such enterprises, because many occupy relatively old buildings, and because few have owners who are familiar with disability and barriers. Another large share will be taken by transportation, although these costs will peak at about 1985 when Transbus is available and many other modifications have already been made. One cost that will be a continuing, as opposed to a one-time, expense is that of providing for communication-barrier removal. Employees must be trained and regularly upgraded in communication skills (fingerspelling, et cetera), while in some cases specialists in communication such as interpreters and readers must be brought in. The funds we spend on research and development, however, should help keep these costs down considerably. This is but one more indication of why we must approach the ten-year plan with a commitment to implement not one or a few of the five points but all five. It does not help to remove barriers to industry if people cannot qualify for work there, obstacles to stores if people cannot afford to shop there, and barriers to colleges if students cannot qualify for admission there.

"Give a man a fish, and he will eat for a day. Teach him how to fish, and he will eat for the rest of his life."

Chinese proverb

4 Reaching for Potential

The December 4, 1977, Philadelphia *Sunday Bulletin* led off with a front-page, four-column, above-the-fold screamer, "Get Rich Quick: Train the Disabled." The story, by Gunter David, a staff reporter, was an exposé of Gerald Schatz's activities as head of educational programs for disabled children in Montgomery County, Pennsylvania. Schatz, the article indicated, had had personal earnings exceeding $458,000 in the 1975–76 school year—all of it paid by the citizens of Pennsylvania. He had placed his wife, his brother, and his son-in-law on the schools' payrolls, again at public expense.

Three days later, the New York *Post* ran a story about a midtown Manhattan school for emotionally disturbed children that had diverted $2.7 million of taxpayers' money to illegal use and had paid its head $77,000 in salary, underwritten his trips to Europe and Morocco, and helped him finance private real-estate ventures. All but three of the school's 292 children were receiving their education at state expense.

Both programs are publicly supported because of state

and federal laws requiring that disabled children be given a public education in local school districts or at private schools at public expense. The intent of the law is to ensure that such children and their parents will have access to education and that parents will not have to pay extra just because their child has a handicap. Prior to these laws, it was not uncommon for parents who could afford it to pay as much as $5,000 to $10,000 each year for private schooling because local schools refused to teach their children.

The Pennsylvania and New York schools, both founded before these laws took effect, accepted state tuition payments—and continued charging the parents. One of Schatz's schools sent parents regular bills for "trips and cookies" and "service fees" totalling as much as $1,000 annually. If the state was late in paying the children's tuition, a common occurrence, the schools merely billed the parents for "temporary" tuition payments. Some parents have had to go to court to get their money back.

Why were such abuses permitted? There seem to be three basic reasons. First, many public school programs, despite state and federal law, continue to refuse to teach disabled children; they merely use more sophisticated reasons for rejection in order to "comply" with the law. Accordingly, because an education is a must, the state must support private education for the children. Second, the state by law can only reimburse expenses at nonprofit educational institutions. What the Pennsylvania and New York schools did was to employ complex bookkeeping, together with huge salaries and generous fringe benefits, to hide the fact that they were making large profits. And they were able to make such profits because of the third reason: the parents did not know of their rights. Desperate to obtain an education for their children, and forced through years of rejection by public schools to pay high costs at private schools, they feared rejection by the private institutions as well if they did not pay, leaving them without recourse— or so they thought. No one was there to advise them of their legal rights and to help them fight the outrageous abuses perpetrated by the schools.

The real tragedy is that, even had they known and fought, the public schools might not have accepted their children. In New York City today, more than nine thousand disabled children have waited six, eight, even twelve months to be admitted into local schools—while more than that number of spaces was already available to accommodate the children on the waiting list. Nationwide, in 1975, as many as 1.75 million disabled children were being denied the education they needed. Even today, with disabled children numbering between 10% and 12% of the school-age population, enrollment of these children in schools averages 7% of the population in school.

A related, though much less scandalous, situation obtains in vocational rehabilitation programming for disabled youths and adults. Of every eleven such persons to qualify for these services, only one is served. The reason has to do not with overt and covert rejection policies, dextrous bookkeeping to disguise obscene profits, or private facilities taking advantage of public-program rejections, but rather with our failure as a nation to invest in rehabilitation. Appropriations from the Congress, together with state-furnished "matching funds," suffice to serve only 9% of the eligible population. With more than four million potential clients in the population as a whole, the annual number of persons rehabilitated each year averages less than three hundred thousand. Partly because of the lack of resources, the federal and state governments have not reached most of the potential beneficiaries with information about available services. Disabled youths and adults, no less than parents of disabled children, remain largely unaware of rights and services to which they are entitled.

These problems are part of a larger one: we have not sought potential in disabled people. We restrict out spending on them in order to "curb costs" and because most of us do not really believe that if we were to invest in disabled people, the investment would bring in any real return to us as a society. That is, we seem not to be convinced that these people can become self-sufficient, independent, taxpaying citizens. The costs we bear because of our failures to invest and to believe have already been documented: they run in the billions annually and are climbing at a rate far outpacing that of the nation's economy.

Consider our spending on education and rehabilitation in comparison with that on disability benefits, insurance, and institutionalization. Whereas the former totals tens of billions of dollars, the latter barely reaches one billion on the federal level in each of these areas. In rehabilitation, for example, federal outlays increased just 3% in 1977, 3% in 1978, 3% in 1979, and are expected to remain virtually at the 1979 level in 1980. At the same time, inflation increased two to three times as fast as increases in rehabilitation funding, thus reducing each year the actual purchasing power of the money. We are cutting back on our real support for rehabilitation at a time when only one out of eleven eligible persons can be served—and when spending on programs whose *raison d'être* comes from our failure to serve the others is rising almost 11% annually. A similar situation occurs in education. In 1975, the Congress pledged to provide 30% of the extra costs of educating disabled children in public programs by 1980, yet actually appropriated only enough to pay 12% of these costs.

The Carter administration's Fiscal Year 1980 Budget offers a few cases in point. It proposes to spend just $218 per child per year on disabled children and wants to provide enough funds to serve only 3.8 million of the nation's disabled children and youth. In rehabilitation, the budget is even more revealing: Carter wants to decrease the number of disabled youths and adults served by ninety thousand and rehabilitate fifteen thousand fewer persons, compared with one year ago.

Both education and rehabilitation for disabled people attract impressive statements of support from the Congress and the administration, as well as in the states. Authorizing legislation proposes bold innovations. Senators and congressmen deliver impassioned speeches on the floor in support of the bills, and vote overwhelmingly for the measures. White House and HEW officials point proudly to their commitment to meet the needs of disabled people. This support, however, is very thin. When the Rehabilitation Act of 1973 was first passed by an overwhelming majority of both houses of Congress, for example, President Nixon's veto was instantly sustained, as legislators did an abrupt flip-flop on the bill. More pointed illustrations can be found by contrasting appropriations bills with authorization measures. The 1975 Education for All Handicapped Children Act, for example, authorized appropriate educational services for "all" eligible children and youth. It contained vigorous, ringing denunciations of policies excluding these children from an education. Yet when the appropriations bill came before the same congressmen and senators, they repeatedly backed down, voting sums which by their very paucity ensured continuation of precisely the same exclusionary practices they had just condemned.

According to the Yankelovich, Skelly, and White survey findings, the American people want more honest support for special efforts on behalf of disabled people. The results of the study indicate that these people believe that barriers must be removed and that "changes that are long overdue" must now be made. The questions before us in the 1980s are whether the general public will sustain its efforts on behalf of these changes, and whether the Congress and the administration will follow its lead. The answers will reveal whether we as a people are ready to invest in disabled people—to teach these people to fish—or are content with nominal gestures and empty promises—with giving disabled people a fish which will last them for only a day.

The Right to an Education

We must begin with an education. Each disabled child must have available to him or her, beginning at the preschool level, opportunities for an appropriate educational program meeting his or her specific needs in the least restrictive environment. The education must be available locally, near the child's home. It is not enough just to place the child in a community school and make available to him or her what is open to other children in the school. Rather, we must ensure that the child's special needs are met, so that he or she will have a chance to benefit from what is available, just as the other children do. It must be a free education.

What I have just said has never been true in the United States. In 1948, only 12% of all disabled children were receiving any special education at all. By 1963, only 21% were being served. The figure in 1967 was 33%. By 1975, 25% (or one in four) were still not being served—and more than half of those who were in some educational setting were not receiving the kinds of assistance they required in order to benefit from the program equally with nondisabled children. By the time of this writing, one child in ten still is not being served. Over a thirty-year period, we have managed to reverse the situation that obtained in 1948. We are making progress, but very slowly. The challenge now is not just to admit these children into programs but to provide them with the kinds of services they need to prepare for life and work.

We have the legislation. The Education for All Handicapped Children Act of 1975 (P.L. 94–142) offers us all the authorization we need to do the job.[1] The act is not the problem. Rather, we have three primary concerns before us now. One, we must put our money where our mouths are: we must appropriate the funds required to implement the 1975 law. Two, we must enforce the requirements on state and local education agencies, preventing them from denying children entrance into schools and from relegating them to inferior education once they are there. Three, we must advise parents and children of their rights, providing them with access to highly trained advocates who can assist them in fighting for their children's rights.

Access. By September 1980, all disabled children aged 3–18 are to have available to them a free appropriate public education. Youths aged 18–21 are to be given the same access prior to September 1981. This access to an education is to be available regardless of the severity of a disability. Whenever possible and when it is in the child's best interests, the education is to be provided locally. Similarly, where the child's needs are best met through instruction in regular classes, mainstreaming into such classes is required. It is important to note that the stress is upon the child's needs and meeting them: if a child will benefit more from a special class within a regular school or even in a special-education facility or institution, such placement is to be provided. The law anticipates that some children will need specialized attention for varying periods, perhaps for several years, or perhaps only for part of a day. It also recognizes that the child's needs may change from time to time and provides that the school must meet those changed needs.

Testing and Evaluation. All instruments used to test or assess a child's skills must be administered in that child's native language or mode of communication (e.g., if a deaf child functions best with sign language and speech together, instructions and other aspects of evaluation must be conducted in those modes). The tests must be the most culture- and bias-free instruments available. Interpretation of results must reflect the guidance of a specialist familiar with the disability, so as to minimize misinterpretations of scores and resulting misdiagnoses and misclassifications.

Due Process. Parents and, when appropriate, the children themselves are to be advised prior to any evaluation of or change in programming for a child; given an opportunity to present complaints about any aspect of the child's program; provided full access to all relevant educational records; granted the opportunity to have an independent assessment done by an evaluation specialist of their own choosing, and at the school's expense, if they are not satisfied with the school's testing program; offered a chance to a due-process hearing before an impartial hearing officer if they do not agree with a school's placement or services; and allowed to appeal any unfavorable decision affecting their child that emerges from such a hearing.

Equal Educational Opportunity. If necessary, a child must be provided with kinds of assistance different from those made available to nondisabled children, if such assistance will help the child obtain the same benefit or the same opportunity for an education. The education must be individualized. P.L. 94–142 places great stress upon such words as "suitable," "appropriate," "designed to develop the maximum potential of," and "specialized" to describe the kinds of opportunities that must be made available for those who could not benefit equally from the same processes and services offered other children. For this reason, the law requires that an "individualized educational program" (IEP) be written for each child, reviewed annually, and revised as appropriate to reflect the child's progress and changed needs. It defines the IEP with these words:

> The term "individualized educational program" means a written statement for each child developed in any meeting by a representative of the local educational agency . . . who shall be qualified to provide, or supervise the provision of, specially designed in-

struction to meet the unique needs of handicapped children, the teacher, the parents or guardian of such child, and whenever appropriate, such child.

The law further defines IEPs by indicating what these plans should include. Five provisions are mandated: (1) a statement of the present levels of educational performance of the child; (2) a statement of annual goals, including short-term instructional objectives; (3) a statement of the specific educational services to be provided to the child, and of the extent to which he or she will participate in regular educational programs; (4) the projected date for initiation of such services and their anticipated duration; and (5) the appropriate objective criteria and evaluation procedures and schedules for determining, on at least an annual basis, whether the instructional objectives are being achieved.

It is unusual for a piece of legislation to be so detailed and explicit. Normally, such specificity is left for the administering federal agency to develop. But in the case of P.L. 94–142, the Congress was determined to protect the rights of children and their parents in the face of overt and blatant denial of these rights in the nation's sixteen thousand school districts.

Vocational Education[2]

The single most blatantly discriminatory aspect of public education for disabled children and youth today is that of vocational education. With 10% to 12% of the school-age population disabled, enrollment in vocational education by disabled youth as a proportion of total vocational education enrollment averages just 1.7%. Of these students, more than 70% are placed, not in the modern facilities made available to nondisabled students, but in separate, segregated, and poorly equipped "special" settings. Yet vocational education is mandatory if disabled youth are to be trained for jobs. Today, a majority of disabled adults of working age is not employed, and, of those who are, earnings average half those of nondisabled workers.

P.L. 94–482, the Amendments to the Vocational Education Act of 1976, requires that 10% of the funds allocated for vocational education be "set aside" to teach disabled youth and that the states "match" that sum with an equal contribution. Disabled students are to be educated with other students whenever possible, and supplementary aids and special education assistance to make mainstreaming successful are provided for in the law. The IEP developed in special education is specifically included in vocational education programming: any vocational education offerings are to be described fully in the student's IEP.

The 1976 law marked a definite departure from previous practices of making vocational education available only to a select portion of the school-age population, the "best" students who needed such preparation for work but did not expect to attain a higher education degree. P.L. 94–482 required access to vocational education for all appropriate students. Yet the administration has consistently refused to support this expansion in scope and has fought, so far successfully, any appropriations to carry out the full-access requirements of the law.

The effect upon disabled youth is disastrous. First, they are denied the training they need to learn how to perform certain specific job functions, and instead are relegated to lower-level "industrial arts" kinds of training, which prepare them, not for employment, but merely for "vocational exploration" or a "taste" of different kinds of careers. Nor is that all. The civil-rights provisions in effect today, notably section 503, which protects applicants and employees in private businesses which carry out government contracts, and section 504, which prohibits discrimination in publicly supported programs and activities, use the term "qualified" to limit the guarantees offered. That is, only "qualified" disabled people are protected. But the restriction in vocational education means that many disabled youths and adults are not eligible for such protection because they are not qualified for the jobs they seek.

Clearly, reform in vocational education for disabled students is urgently needed. This fact becomes even more apparent when the range of vocational education offerings is considered. The law defines vocational education as organized educational programs which are directly related to the preparation of individuals for paid or unpaid employment, or for additional preparation for a career requiring other than a baccalaureate or advanced degree. It includes secondary, post-secondary, and adult education and is generally delivered through several "cluster areas," including agricultural education, business and office education, consumer and homemaking education, distributive education, industrial arts education, trade and industrial education, and diversified cooperative education. Some of these terms require a little explanation. "Distributive" education concerns marketing and distribution of products, while "diversified cooperative education" offers work opportunities in addition to classroom study. Vocational education, then, is that part of education that makes an individual more employable in one group of occupations than another, as opposed to more fundamental kinds of instruction which seek only to offer pre-vocational or "introduction-to-the-world-of-work" kinds of experiences.

Can we accomplish such reform? Can the entire range of vocational education be opened for disabled students, even those with the most severe handicaps? Happily, the answer is yes. Consider the case of Special Intermediate School District 916 in White Bear Lake, Minnesota. What makes the difference in this school district is the attitude of Superintendent William Knack. He is committed to serving disabled students in all phases of the district's impressive program, which enrolls 1,100 high-school seniors, 1,800 post-secondary-level adults, and 5,500 part-time or extension students. Among those served are 400 trainable mentally retarded students, preschool through adult.

At White Bear Lake, there are no "special" or segregated services: virtually everything the school does is done in an integrated fashion, with support services available for those who need them. The stress is upon self-directed, individualized instruction. So successful is the self-paced approach that 70% of the students graduate without requiring special assistance in their classes.

One of the most exciting potential uses of vocational education lies in preparing the "young old" for rewarding careers following retirement. With more and more people retiring as early as age fifty-five, and with longevity giving persons who reach age sixty-five an average of sixteen additional years of life, we now have a relatively healthy, capable population of people aged 55–75 who may desire to continue working or at least to remain productive and contribute to the community. Vocational education, through adult and continuing education classes, can prepare these people for a broad range of jobs and voluntary contributions.

Traditionally, both medical and educational leaders have dismissed the over-fifty-five population. Vocational rehabilitation, for example, rarely accepts persons over the age of fifty-four for evaluation, training, and placement. The attitude has been "concentrate upon those who have a full life ahead of them, not upon these people who will die soon." This attitude has always been unfortunate, but today it is indefensible. A fifty-five-year-old may very well work for another fifteen years, certainly long enough for society to recoup its investment in his or her training, and at the same time he or she may live and contribute to the community for at least twenty years even if employment is not sought. Either way, we must invest in the resources of these people.

Dr. Marc Gold has worked in Dixon State Hospital and the University of Illinois with severely mentally retarded individuals to develop what he calls his "Try Another Way" approach to teaching retarded persons complex vocational tasks. Gold's method is simplicity itself: the task is broken down into small, manageable components, each of which is taught until it is mastered. As he puts it: "If these people don't learn, it's the result of our incompetence—not theirs." His films are helping to convince other vocational educators to adopt similar techniques.

Perhaps the most difficult aspect of reforming vocational education is ridding its teachers and administrators of their stereotyped notions about what disabled and elderly people can do. Most vocational educators are trained not so much in education or other helping fields as in the vocational area itself. That is, they are people who have worked for many years as repairmen, technicians, engineers, and small businessmen. Large numbers literally do not know about the vast range of occupations in which disabled and elderly people now work—and no one, not federal administrators, not state agency representatives, not local school board members, is telling them about this. As a result, they frequently reject disabled and old students from their classes and, if they do teach these persons, teach only the more traditional skills: deaf people are trained to become printers ("because the noise of the machines won't bother them"), blind people are actually taught basket weaving. It would be funny if it were not so tragic.

Career Education

Beginning as early as kindergarten and continuing virtually throughout life, career education is designed to offer career awareness, career exploration, and career preparation. It is not a series of classes or courses; rather, career education is expected to "infuse," or be an integral part of, other educational activities. Thus, a ninth-grade English class offering information about and exploration of such fields as journalism, the teaching of English, and other English-related careers is engaging in career education. The U.S. Office of Education defines it as "the totality of experiences through which one learns about and prepares to engage in work as part of his or her way of living."

For disabled children, career education can mean being exposed to and learning to identify stereotyping in employment patterns. Such stereotyping is so pervasive that often the disabled individual is not even aware of it: he or she has been surrounded by it since birth or very early in life. Accordingly, the disabled child and youth tends to blame not the people who stereotype, but himself or herself, and to seek not the kinds of jobs he or she would enjoy and be good at but the jobs "people like me do."

A personal example may be helpful. The author struggled through twenty-two years of life without even the vaguest idea of what a deaf person was supposed to do. I liked writing and wanted more than anything else to be an investigative reporter for a newspaper. The problem was that investigative reporting by definition is reporting based upon what no one has written before: the reporter gathers his facts *de novo,* as it were, through interviews and telephone conversations. Because I was deaf, I could not imagine a way of doing this, and accordingly ruled it out automatically. Today, the work I do as director of the American Coalition of Citizens with Disabilities (ACCD), the national advocate for disabled people, is almost precisely what I would do as an investigative reporter. I find out what is happening and what might happen to affect disabled people and write about it. The difference is that I know now that my deafness does not stop me from doing investigative reporting. I have found ways of getting around the disability, and I understand now that what matters is what I can do, my talents and abilities, rather than what I can't do. That it took me more than two decades to discover this provides an indication of just how potent are stereotyped notions about disability in America—and how deeply these affect the disabled person's self-concept and career aspirations.

Career education for disabled students can also mean very much what it means for other students: awareness of possible careers, the requirements of entry into each, and the kinds of opportunities each offers for self-fulfillment and financial support. An excellent way of doing this is to help the students meet disabled adults in the community who are performing a wide range of jobs, get to know not only how these people do their work but also how their careers affect and are affected by their lifestyles, and come to understand what they themselves, as people with handicaps, might enjoy doing and might do well.

One other benefit of career education for disabled as well as nondisabled students is that it often increases motivation to excel in academic subjects such as English, mathematics, and science. Students learn just how important writing, speaking, calculating, reasoning, and investigating are to success in many occupations and accordingly appreciate more than they might otherwise just how valuable these "boring" subjects are and how relevant to their own lives and hopes.

How can we implement career education for disabled persons? By reviewing our curricula and other organized educational activities and, when necessary, supplementing them with appropriate career-related instruction. We can do this through four phases of a person's development:

Career Awareness (kindergarten to fifth grade). Intended to stimulate the child's interest in and awareness of work as it relates to the self, the home, the family, and the community, the awareness phase begins in kindergarten (or even earlier) and extends through the fifth grade. For disabled children, the stress must be on what people with these disabilities do, particularly on the vast range of occupations such persons have already succeeded in, so as to dispel stereotyped notions of career limitations.

Career Orientation (6–7). The emphasis in this phase is not only on what is possible for the child but more narrowly on what this child himself or herself wants to do and be. Thus, the child relates knowledge about himself or herself with the requirements and expectations of different fields.

Career Exploration (8–9). This phase is one of prevocational training, that is, exposure to different tools, terminology, and basic skills. Included is a series of tests and other evaluation instruments and procedures helping the student to identify the specific kinds of capacities he or she will need in a certain cluster of occupations and helping the student to develop these skills.

Career Preparation (10-A). The final phase may extend into early and even late adulthood. It might involve specific vocational education, higher education, and even paid employment. Its aim is to offer opportunities for developing the skills needed for specific career areas, including advancement to higher-level jobs and mid-life career changes.

We must not wait until high-school or post-secondary levels to begin helping disabled children and youth to learn about what they can do for the rest of their lives. This, briefly, is why career education forms a vital part of our nation's agenda helping disabled people out of dependence and into independence.

Vocational Rehabilitation

One of the most exciting ventures into which the federal government has entered since the turn of the century is the federal-state partnership in vocational rehabilitation. Begun in the early 1920s as, in part, a reaction to the casualties of World War I, vocational rehabilitation has demonstrated that it returns more than nine dollars to the federal treasury for every dollar expended. People who previously were unemployed have been trained and placed in jobs, moving from being tax-users to tax-payers. In fact, the nine-to-one ratio of return on investment is conservative, because it leaves out state taxes, social-security taxes, sales taxes, and other payments to government, as well as stimulation of the economy generally when people have money they can and do spend in the community. Rehabilitation does not cost, it pays.

In a series of five columns published in 1976, Sylvia Porter, the highly respected economist, explored the cost-benefit figures of rehabilitation spending. Calling the return of nine dollars on every dollar spent "awesome," she attacked the "unbelievable, unqualified negativism" of the federal government in refusing to increase its support for rehabilitation. Porter used terms like "astounding," "spectacular economic return," "truly magnificent," and other superlatives to describe rehabilitation's economic benefits, while she lambasted the administration for opposing expansion of the program.[3]

What is the program that attracts such praise and yet elicits what Porter calls "non-support" and "non-execution of the law" from the federal government? The vocational rehabilitation program represents a partnership between the federal government, which pays more than three-fourths of the costs, and the states in which persons who are disabled receive evaluation, diagnosis, counseling, vocational training, and placement services. The effort aims to develop the potential of the person and help him or her overcome the effects of the disability. It is a goal-oriented program.

For reasons that remain obscure, federal administrators, particularly the White House's Office of Management and Budget, persist in confusing rehabilitation with welfare. The objective, they contend, is to "control" and "manage" expenditures, producing savings in the budget. This "tomorrow morning" economic thinking ignores the return on investment in rehabilitation and actually costs the federal government billions of dollars. Presidents Richard Nixon, Gerald Ford, and Jimmy Carter, all preoccupied with inflation and reducing federal expenditures, have all made the same tragic mistakes. Each fought for cuts and restraints in the program.

In 1978, for example, the states were prepared to "match"—that is, put up their share of—as much as $947 million. The Carter administration fought the states for six full months, seeking an authorization level that represented virtually no increase over the previous year. In 1979, the states would have been able to match well over $1 billion in federal funds, yet once again Carter resisted, asking for precisely the same amount as had been appropriated the year before. In 1980, the pattern was repeated. This from a president who campaigned with the pledge to increase rehabilitation spending "substantially."

The nation's governors in recent years have formed an

even more serious threat to the program. Incensed at Washington's tendency to enact programs for which the federal government would provide part, but not all, of the funds, the National Governors Association called for federal assumption of the entire cost of new programs involving state and local governments. It passed at its Boston meeting in the summer of 1978 a resolution introduced by California Governor Jerry Brown, who called it "the real Truth in Spending Act," insisting that any new federal-state programs be funded entirely from Washington.[4]

It is difficult to imagine any proposal which would be more devastating to service programs for disabled children, youths, and adults. The states traditionally have had the responsibility to provide these services. In fact, it is only in recent years that the federal government got involved in education for disabled children at all. But when it did, it understandably wanted some control over how the monies were spent. The legislation and the accompanying regulations have spelled out, in increasingly specific detail, the expectation of the federal government that the rights of disabled people be protected and that the services made possible by these federal funds not be denied to any disabled individual. Were the federal government to pay all of the costs of the programs, this tendency would go to its ultimate degree: the federal government, not the states, would be providing the services. Such an abdication of responsibility by the states would be reprehensible and, one would hope, not exactly what the governors had in mind when they endorsed Brown's resolution urging the president to ask for and the Congress to pass a law which would "require the federal government to reimburse state and local governments for the full cost of implementing congressional and executive directives, including new programs, increased service requirements, and revenue losses."

That same summer, the governors and the administration combined to very nearly defeat the attempt of the Congress to amend and extend the Rehabilitation Act of 1973. It was only due to the courageous defense of the program by the state rehabilitation agencies, disabled people, and the congressional authorizing committees that the Rehabilitation, Comprehensive Services, and Developmental Disabilities Amendment of 1978 became law. Stung by the enactment, the administration, particularly the Office of Management and Budget and HEW, promptly began preparing for what it called "perfecting amendments" and what the rest of us would refer to as "gutting the law." First, the administration proposed appropriations far below those authorized by the Congress; independent living for severely disabled people, to take just one example, was authorized at $80 million and the administration proposed just $2 million. Then, HEW and the Office of Management and Budget submitted proposals to revise the law itself. The administration's opposition to spending money on rehabilitation became so pronounced that syndicated columnist Jack Anderson went on national television and wrote a special column warning of the coming raids on the program.[5]

The federal opposition stands in sharp contrast with the support of many states. California, for example, has for several years invested much more than its share of money in the program. Arkansas, responding to the fact that it has the nation's highest per-capita rate of disability, is another strong leader. Recently, however, the efforts of the governors to cut state budgets have curtailed the progress of these and other state agencies. The situation in the states between the governors and the program managers parallels closely that in Washington between the administration and the Congress. There can be no question that state and federal administrators must be helped to understand the program better and to realize how self-defeating their opposition to rehabilitation spending is.

Beyond that, we must seek to implement the 1978 law fully. This landmark piece of legislation offers for the first time important services for disabled persons who do not have an immediate potential for paid employment but who can be helped to more independent living through the provision of counseling, supportive services, attendant care, information and referral programs, and related services. It also extends the basic state-federal partnership, expands the research program, and provides for innovative job-creation efforts in community employment.

Independent Living. P.L. 95–602 establishes, in Title VII, a program of "comprehensive services for independent living" that is "designed to meet the current and future needs of individuals whose disabilities are so severe that they do not presently have the potential for employment but who may benefit from vocational rehabilitation services which will enable them to live and function independently." Priority is to be given to persons not served under the traditional work-oriented program.

What is involved in independent living? The act suggests counseling services, including psychological, psychotherapeutic, and related services; housing, including modifications and accommodations of any space to serve disabled persons, which assists in more independence; job placement services, as appropriate; transportation; attendant care; physical rehabilitation, including medical restoration of capacity or improvement in functioning; prostheses and other appliances and devices; health maintenance; recreational activities; services for children of preschool age, including physical therapy, development of language and communication skills, and child-development services; and appropriate preventive services to decrease the needs of disabled individuals for rehabilitation services in the future. This broad range of activities is intended to ensure that barriers, obstacles, and other hindrances to independence are removed, so the person may develop his or her capacities and interests, reducing dependence on the family and on public support through social security, welfare, and income maintenance. At the same time, the program moves people inexorably toward employment as an ultimate rather than an immediate goal. Persons served with independent-living funds typically will require several years of assistance before they are prepared to begin formal vocational training, if indeed they ever are.

So important did the Congress regard independent living as being that it authorized payment by the federal government of 90% of the costs of the program. The states may put up their 10% matching share "in kind," if they desire, by, for example, contributing manpower, space, or other services, and need not match with actual tax-revenue dollars. The Congress also provided that no state, no matter how small, would receive less than $200,000 annually for carrying out the program. These unusual steps make it as easy as possible for the state governments to implement independent living. Contrasted with the regular vocational rehabilitation program, the federal share is significantly larger. Even more vivid is the contrast with federal support of education for disabled children and youth. In education, the federal share currently is only 12% of the extra costs of teaching disabled children, with the states and localities putting up 88%. There can be no question of Congress's commitment to the program. This investment is well spent, because independent-living services directly attack the huge and escalating dependence costs incurred on behalf of severely disabled persons who must rely on social security and welfare to survive.

One important part of the new program is support for what are called "centers for independent living." These programs, the most famous of which is the Berkeley, California, Center for Independent Living (CIL), have for several years had to struggle mightily to scrounge funds to support their work. It has become a necessity at CIL, for example, to devote considerable effort just to raising money. The centers have had to qualify for and apply to local, state, and federal agencies, foundations, corporations, and other sources of funding. CIL receives support from rehabilitation, community-development, Title XX social-service, employment-training, research, and transportation programs. What P.L. 95–602 established was a single source of support for programs like CIL, so that these facilities would have at least one continuing source of revenue upon which they could depend.

In creating this program, the act recognized that the independent-living movement is as much an effort by disabled people themselves as it is by professionals serving this population. Any applicant for independent-living-center funds must demonstrate that disabled individuals will be "substantially involved in policy direction and management" and will be employed by the center. The scope of services envisioned by the act in centers for independent living is broad. It includes counseling, training in jobseeking skills, assistance in using equipment and devices needed because of the disability, housing-referral and related services, transportation, the development of directories of services within the community that are accessible to, and needed by, disabled people, education for living independently in the community (including money management, legal rights as a tenant, consumer-affairs and similar training), social and recreational activities, attendant care and the training of attendants, and "such other services as may be necessary."

Knowing that so broad a range of essential services would be costly to provide and that the return on the investment would be more delayed than is the case with direct-employment services, the Congress authorized $80 million for the first year (1979), $150 million for the second year, and $200 million for the third year, with "such sums as may be necessary" for the fourth year. These sums are not as large as they might at first appear. Independent living is to be administered by state rehabilitation agencies, of which there are eighty-four in the country, including many specifically for blind persons and several in trust territories and islands administered by the United States. Thus, the average first-year authorization would be $950,000 per agency (more for the larger agencies, no less than $200,000 for the smaller states), or enough to serve perhaps nine hundred people in each agency. The nationwide total would be 75,600 persons served, a relatively modest beginning when one considers that there are several millions who need assistance. By contrast, the administration's proposal of $2 million for the program would serve only twenty-five persons per agency at $24,000 to an average-sized agency, or 2,100 persons nationwide. These figures exemplify vividly the complete inadequacy of the administration's plan.

Basic State Services. P.L. 95–602 authorizes a total of $808 million for the traditional rehabilitation program in Fiscal Year 1979. For succeeding years, the sum is to be increased by a cost-of-living factor but is not to exceed $880 million in 1980, $945 million in 1981, and $972 million in 1982. The administration is seeking to appeal the cost-of-living factor and has proposed that the 1979 figure be continued virtually without increase in 1980. Under its plan, thousands fewer than those persons now served would be helped, in an era when rehabilitation has funding only to serve one out of every eleven eligible individuals. And because inflation cuts the purchasing power of each rehabilitation dollar, the quality of services would be impaired. If the cost-of-living formula were repealed, the situation would grow more serious with each passing year.

The basic state-services program offers diagnosis and evaluation to persons who apply for assistance, helping them and their counselors to determine whether they have a vocational potential and if so in what kinds of careers. Equipment and devices such as hearing aids, wheelchairs, and canes may be provided; if the individual is able to afford it, he or she pays part of the cost. Individual and group counseling are made available, and training in specific job areas is offered. Finally, the agency will help the person obtain a job commensurate with his or her abilities and training, and will follow up to ensure that the placement is appropriate and that any additional services required are delivered.

Each client has the right to participate in the writing

of his or her own "individual written rehabilitation program" (IWRP), which is in many respects similar to the IEP in education. In fact, as the disabled person moves from school to rehabilitation, the IEP and IWRP are to be written in conjunction to ensure an orderly transition in services. The IWRP states the vocational objective, together with the sequence of services to be provided and the extent to which the individual will participate in financing services. If the client disagrees with the plan suggested by his or her counselor, an appeal is possible and the plan may be rewritten.

Extensive studies have documented the cost-benefit return on investment in the program. Abt Associates in Boston, Berkeley Planning Associates, and other consulting firms have traced, in exhaustive detail, just how remarkably effective the program is. The Berkeley study, for example, found a return of $16 for every dollar invested; among the more severely disabled, who are usually more expensive to serve, the return was a healthy $9.13. Despite these facts, increases in funding have fallen far short of the inflation rate, producing a decline since the mid-seventies in numbers of persons served and rehabilitated.

Research. The 1978 act took a bold step forward in the area of research on prevention, cure, amelioration, and rehabilitation of disability. Noting that a plethora of small research programs was scattered across government, the U.S. House of Representatives Committee on Science and Technology convened a Panel on Research Programs to Aid the Handicapped. The panel met for six months in 1976 and was convened again for another six months in 1977. Its report recommended the creation of a consolidated research institute and the formation of a council of government officials, private researchers, and disabled persons to oversee the institute's program. Olin E. ("Tiger") Teague, the Texas Democrat who chaired the committee, deserves much of the credit for the fact that the institute-council formula was enthusiastically adopted by the House Committee on Education and Labor, which wrote it almost without change into P.L. 95–602.

Section 202 of this law establishes a National Institute of Handicapped Research, which is to be headed by a director appointed by the president. So important did the Congress regard the institute that it waived the usual civil-service red-tape requirements for employment of top-level staff members of the institute and established unusually high levels of compensation for the director and deputy director. The institute is to administer the nation's rehabilitation-research and training-center program, coordinate federal efforts relating to research in rehabilitation, disseminate information and materials produced by research programs and activities, and produce regular reports on the health, income, and other characteristics of the country's population of thirty-six million disabled persons.

Title IV of the act creates a National Council on the Handicapped, whose fifteen members are to include at least five disabled individuals, as well as researchers, rehabilitation professionals, business, and labor. The council, which meets at least quarterly and has its own staff, is responsible for establishing general policies for the institute as well as for advising the commissioner of Rehabilitation Services about rehabilitation and independent-living programs. It is to conduct systematic reviews of all programs and policies conducted by the federal government on behalf of disabled people, reporting regularly to the president and the Congress.

The National Council provides, for the first time, a high-level, responsible forum in which experts in rehabilitation and research, as well as disabled persons themselves, may directly influence federal policy affecting disabled people. It is important as well because it provides a central coordinating body which can take a comprehensive look at the entire range of programs and activities relating to disability, ensuring that gaps and duplications are eliminated and that scarce resources are directed and targeted toward the most crucial needs.

The Congress authorized $50 million in Fiscal Year 1979 for the institute, with the amount rising to $75 million in 1980, $90 million in 1981, and $100 million in 1982. For the council, the act provides in each year "such sums as may be necessary" to carry out its responsibilities. As is the case with independent living and basic state services, the administration has resisted investing in research. It has proposed that the 1979 figure of $31.5 million be retained as under current appropriations rather than increased to $50 million and has asked that 1980 spending be reduced to $27.5 million. The effect of these proposals can readily be appreciated when it is considered that the $27.5 million sum is less than was spent a full decade ago on rehabilitation research and that the effect of inflation over that period has halved the purchasing power of these dollars. Thus the administration wants to spend, in real terms, only 50% of what was spent in 1969, despite the fact that the new law expands considerably the responsibility of the federal government in research and development activities.

Employment. P.L. 95–602 creates, in Title VI, a community-service employment program for disabled persons who are not now working. The initiative, to be administered by the Department of Labor, contains some exciting innovations. First, attendants, readers, and interpreters needed to enable disabled persons to work effectively may be employed under the program, at no cost to the individual or the organization hiring him or her. Second, as an incentive to work, the law permits disabled persons now on dependence rolls such as Medicaid to continue receiving protection under these programs despite the fact of employment. The threat of cutoffs in benefits, with the attendant two-year wait before eligibility can be restored, is a major disincentive to employment for many severely disabled persons. Third, the act prohibits pay levels for the disabled employees that are below those provided for nondisabled persons performing the same tasks. Fourth, the projects may pay the transportation expenses disabled people incur coming to and from work, insofar as these exceed those encountered by nondisabled individuals, as well as other work-related expenses. These provisions are important because it is often more expensive for a disabled person to work than it is for others, thus producing a situation in which the disabled individual's real take-home pay is less.

The Congress authorized $35 million for Fiscal Year 1979, $50 million for 1980, $75 million for 1981, and $100 million for 1982 to cover the 90% share of the program which is to be borne by the federal government. The funds are sufficient only for a pilot program in selected communities, but this is what the Congress intended. It wanted to test the innovations before moving to a broader-based program. The administration, however, wants to cut the support to just $10 million per year.

Developmental Disabilities. P.L. 95–602 amends, not only the Rehabilitation Act of 1973, but also the Developmental Disabilities Services and Facilities Construction Act of 1970. The new law defines "developmental disabilities" to include severe disabilities which occur prior to the age of twenty-two, are likely to continue indefinitely, result in substantial functional limitations in several key areas (e.g., self-care, language, mobility, capacity for independent living, and economic self-sufficiency), and reflect the person's need for a combination of special services which are of extended or lifelong duration and are individually coordinated and planned. The term, then, refers to persons who become disabled very early in life and, as a result of their impairments, need to have a sequence of specialized services provided over a long period of time. The act repealed the previous definition, which restricted eligibility to persons who have mental retardation, cerebral palsy, epilepsy, or autism.

Title V of the act basically continues the previously authorized program, including protection and advocacy systems on behalf of developmentally disabled persons, research and training, and development of state plans for service delivery. The law also authorizes provision of services to developmentally disabled individuals which may be expected to help them become more self-sufficient. Support for these activities remains relatively constant. Despite the lack of increases in authorized funding, the program can at least expect to get appropriations close to what was authorized because the administration has not asked for large cuts.

Meeting the Challenge:
Education and Rehabilitation

It is in reaching for potential that we must make our most significant investment, for it is here that we are directly helping people out of dependence and into independence. Support for education and rehabilitation has been manifestly inadequate for decades and we are paying the price for our negligence in dependence costs that threaten to run out of control. We cannot halt this spiral and then reverse it without making it possible for disabled and elderly people to escape or leave welfare, social-security, and income-maintenance rolls. Our best bets for doing this are education and rehabilitation. Moreover, both programs have proven records of paying rather than costing. The resulting income taxes paid to the federal treasury alone exceed the sums invested in these programs. And with so many not now being served or receiving only some of the assistance they need, the programs are ready for real increases in levels of support.

As part of the ten-year, five-point $22 billion-a-year plan, I suggest spending a total of $184 billion over the coming decade on the federal, state, local, and private levels. This new spending would enable us to reach and help those not now being served adequately. The costs would be shared by the four sectors according to existing patterns. Thus, the federal share of education costs would be that authorized by the 1975 Education for All Handicapped Children Act (30%, in 1981, 40% in 1982 and beyond); the federal government is now appropriating only enough to support 12% in 1981. It must increase its investment and keep its commitment to the states. In rehabilitation, the share appropriated matches that authorized, so the ratio would not be affected by these proposals.

Spending on education for disabled children now approximates $9 billion annually, of which the federal government provides $1 billion (12%) and the states $8 billion. Were the federal share that which has been authorized, the spending would be $2.7 billion on the federal level and $6.3 billion on the state level. I am proposing on the average over the coming decade that $6 billion on the federal level be provided and $9 billion on the state level in new funds. In rehabilitation, current spending is about $1.3 billion, of which the federal share is $1 billion and the states match $0.3 billion. I am proposing that we provide sufficient funds to serve eligible disabled people. New federal spending would average $9 billion and state expenditures $3 billion annually. Private spending would increase much more slowly. Of course, averages are misleading. In human-service programs, it is necessary to permit the states sufficient time to absorb new funds. Accordingly, the proposed increases will rise gradually until 1984, at which point they would maintain a four-year plateau and then begin to fall. The decline reflects the expectation that by 1985 rehabilitation will have eliminated its huge backlog of cases and have begun concentrating on new cases, while many disabled children will have come into the system at earlier ages than in the past, thus needing fewer specialized services from both education and rehabilitation. The decline is not as steep as might be expected because it will be necessary to provide assistance to "young old" disabled persons, those aged 55–75, who desire and need vocational education and rehabilitation services in order to work or contribute to the community. This population will increase markedly from now to 2030. Between 25% and 35% are expected to be disabled, slightly more than at present, but it is difficult to project the numbers that will request education and rehabilitation services.

Specifically, I feel we will need to spend $10 billion in new funds in 1981, $15 billion in 1982, $19 billion in 1983, $22 billion in 1984–87, $20 billion in 1988, $18 billion in 1989, and $14 billion in 1990.

The return on this investment may be expected to exceed $1.6 trillion, based upon conservative calculations. Impressive as this figure might be, the more exciting result, for me, is the provision to every disabled American of an opportunity to help himself or herself achieve to limits defined not by disabilities but by abilities—to achieve "independence and self-confidence, the feeling of creativity, . . . lives of high spirits rather than hushed, suffocating silence."

"Human rights are not conditional. And a commitment to a conditional human right is no commitment at all."

Edward M. Kennedy[1]

5 Dependence and Independence

Historically, we as a nation have perceived disabled and elderly people as individuals deserving of some kind of protection and care. We have not seen them as persons who could and should become self-sufficient. The caretaker philosophy may have been appropriate at times in the past when our nation did not have the capability to help these persons overcome the effects of their disabilities. Today, however, we do have that capability: it is possible for virtually every disabled person who is at least minimally alert and who has some degree of mobility, even if only of a severely restricted kind, to work. Of the sixteen million noninstitutionalized disabled persons of working age, perhaps as many as fifteen million are potentially employable. They, like millions of persons over 55 years of age, can become independent, self-sufficient tax-payers.

This should not be surprising. People with disabilities and senior citizens are also persons with abilities. A person's potential for work is, or should be, less a factor of the disability than of the ability; that is, how far up a career ladder a particular individual goes depends more upon his or her intelligence, drive, skills and talents, training, and other capabilities than upon a disability. Stated differently, when the disability is controlled through accommodations, barrier removal, special devices, and other measures, an individual's potential is what it would be without the disability.

Yet a majority of disabled people today is not working, One important reason may be found in the nature and structure of dependence-oriented programs. We will examine two such programs in this chapter—Social Security Disability Insurance (SSDI) and Supplemental Security Income (SSI). Reforming these programs will not in itself remove the underlying causes of dependence among disabled and elderly people, but it will contribute markedly toward that goal. And, done in conjunction with steps proposed in other chapters, reform will help us to rehabilitate not only disabled and elderly people but America itself.

SSDI: A Program in Crisis

The Social Security Disability Insurance (SSDI) program was created in 1956 to offer protection to workers against the devastating effects of a long-term disability. By 1965, it was still a relatively small program, paying out $1.5 billion annually to fewer than one million beneficiaries. By 1978, however, more than five million beneficiaries and their dependents were receiving $13 billion in benefits. The cost of the program had increased sixteenfold in twenty years. Over the past ten years alone, costs rose 500%. By 1985, the cost is expected to hit $27 billion— with no end in sight.

The program is financed through a payroll tax. When it was first created, employees and employers each contributed 0.250% of taxable earnings up to a maximum taxable amount of $4,400; self-employed individuals were taxed at a rate of 0.375% of earnings up to the maximum taxable amount. In 1966, the maximum taxable income was raised to $6,600 and the employee/employer contribution rate to 0.350%. The figures were raised again in 1968, 1970, 1972, and each succeeding year through 1977. The Social Security Amendments of 1977 increased the maximum taxable amount to $17,700, beginning in 1978, with employees and employers each contributing 0.775% and self-employed persons 1.090%. By 1981, the ceiling amount is expected to be $29,900. It will increase to $42,600 in 1984 if inflation continues as anticipated. By 1990, the tax rate for employees and employers will rise to 1.10% and that for self-employed persons will be 1.65%.

The taxes are deposited in the disability-insurance trust fund, and it is from this fund that monthly benefits are paid to eligible persons and their dependents. About 95% of all persons employed in the United States contribute to the fund. More than eighty million workers are potentially eligible for benefits if they become disabled.

Each year, 1.2 million people apply for benefits. Of these, approximately 60% are denied eligibility. Many of those rejected, as well as many accepted but given benefits lower than they had expected, appeal the decision. HEW must employ six hundred administrative law judges (more than the number of judges in the entire federal court system) to review the cases and even so a backlog of eighteen thousand cases exists, creating a seven-month waiting period for each new case.

The average benefit received monthly by those on the rolls is $319. With the poverty line at $360 per month, that is not a particularly high level of benefits. And the system uses the most stringent definition of disability employed by any program serving disabled people—the applicant must be so totally disabled as to be unable to perform any work anywhere in the national economy. Yet, the numbers served have increased rapidly—2 million in 1967, 2.6 million in 1970, 3.4 million in 1973, 4.5 million in 1976, and the costs have spiralled from $1.8 billion in 1967 to $9 billion in 1976. In fact, had the 1977 social-security legislation not been enacted, the SSDI trust fund would have gone bankrupt early in 1980.[2]

Dramatic as these cost increases are, the problems besetting the SSDI program do not end there. One of the most tragic aspects of the program is that it actually discourages disabled and elderly individuals from seeking and obtaining work. The disincentives, together with our country's failure to invest adequately in rehabilitation, prevent all but 1.5% of SSDI beneficiaries from returning to work. The beginnings of these problems may be seen in the development in 1948 of a concept known as "substantial gainful activity."

THE SGA LIMIT

In 1948, the Advisory Committee on Social Security recommended to the Senate that eligibility for an insurance program for disabled people be limited to people whose disability is one "which is medically demonstrable by objective tests, which prevents the worker from performing any substantial gainful activity, and which is likely to be of long continued and indefinite duration." The Congress, in its Social Security Amendments of 1954, adopted strikingly similar language: disability was defined as the "inability to engage in any substantial gainful activity because of any medically determinable physical or mental impairment that can be expected to be of long continued and indefinite duration." Eligibility was further restricted to those who had shown, very recently, a "substantial" ability to work; this was defined as employment in covered work during at least twenty of the preceding forty quarters.

What was meant by "inability to engage in substantial gainful activity" (SGA)? The Congress left this question for administrative determination by the executive branch. The Social Security Administration set SGA at $100 per month in 1965, increasing it to $125 in 1966 and 1967, $140 between 1968 and 1973, $200 between 1974 and 1978, and $240 beginning in 1978. Thus, an individual who can earn as much as $240 per month, or $120 less than the official poverty level, is not considered to be disabled and is denied eligibility for SSDI.

Why was the level set so low? The legislative history behind the social-security acts indicates that the Congress intended the program to serve only those persons who were "totally" disabled; that is, unable to work at all. And the regulations governing the SSDI program provide that if a beneficiary proves capable of earning more than $50 a month for nine months (not necessarily consecutive) he or she is considered no longer disabled and is removed from the rolls.

Given the low level of benefits and the likelihood of removal from the rolls after such modest earnings, why do so many disabled individuals apply for SSDI benefits?

The answer lies in the "extras" made available subsequent to the determination of SSDI eligibility. Medicare, for example, is extended to beneficiaries who have been on the rolls for two years. Many disabled persons could not afford the medical care offered under this program even if they earned as much as $15,000 a year; equally important, employment is often tentative, subject to abrupt termination, whereas Medicare coverage continues unabated so long as eligibility remains.

But there is another side to this. The low level of SGA constitutes a powerful disincentive to employment. Consider, for example, the instance of an individual who earns more than $50 a month for ten months. In the tenth month, he faces a tax rate of more than 100% on his earnings. Assume a benefit level of $300 per month and earnings of $250 after taxes. In the ninth month, the net monthly income was $550; the following (tenth) month, the net income drops $300 for an effective tax rate of 120%. This is in addition to the loss of Medicare coverage. Understandably, many disabled persons consider that a high price to pay for resuming employment—particularly in light of the fact that should employment be terminated, a two-year waiting period must be endured before eligibility can be re-established—two years without any benefits or Medicare coverage. What many beneficiaries do is to work while receiving SSDI benefits, but to restrict earnings to less than the SGA limit. Perhaps as many as 25% of all beneficiaries are working at any given time. Earnings below $50 per month, however, barely bring income up to the poverty level. The result is a classic "Catch-22" situation—disabled persons who stay on the rolls earn too little to live even at poverty levels, yet those who leave the rolls fare even worse.

The frustrations encountered by disabled individuals can be illustrated in the case of Tom Brown (not his real name). Let us consider how Tom attempted to meet the expenses required for survival and at the same time satisfy his need to perform satisfying work.

TOM BROWN: A CASE HISTORY

Tom was involved in an accident in April 1963 that left him severely disabled. A quadriplegic (unable to control voluntarily hands, arms, feet, and legs, and paralyzed from the neck down), Tom uses an electric wheelchair costing $1,900. For many people, so severe a disability, with its devastating effects upon the ability even to perform mundane, everyday activities, would be crushing. Tom, however, returned to college and obtained a B.S. from a major university in 1971. For six months, he sought a job in vain.

His first job lasted nine months. A second was ended after five months when the company relocated and Tom was unable to move to the new city. In November 1973, he got a third job as an engineer. Tom's gross earnings in this job were $1,091 per month. This unprecedented level of earnings resulted in the determination by the Social Security Administration (SSA) that he was "no longer disabled." In January 1974, all benefits and medical coverage ended.

The determination was devastating for Tom. In addition to the wheelchair he needed, he also had to pay for a specially equipped van costing $10,000 and extraordinary medical expenses arising from his disability (an average of $500 per month), in addition to the usual costs incurred by most persons who work. Tom's real take-home pay, after these disability-related costs, was only $97 per month. He had to pay for food, lodging, transportation to and from work, and incidental expenses out of this modest amount.

Tom fought the SSA decision for three years, taking his case before four different courts. Finally, in April 1977, an administrative-law judge ruled that the "extraordinary" expenses Tom incurred because of his work could be discounted against the SGA limit and that he was therefore entitled to receive benefits from SSDI. His was the first case in which such costs were allowed.

What is perhaps most interesting about Tom Brown is that he refused to permit his disability to make him dependent upon others. He wanted to work, so much so that he endured hardships most workers cannot even imagine. Yet Tom is not unique: thousands of disabled persons daily face similar hardships and insist upon resolving their problems independently. The tragedy is that so few of them are given even a remotely fair chance.

REFORMING SSDI

Removing the disincentives to employment that now characterize the SSDI program would provide a major boost to rehabilitating disabled and elderly people, particularly when combined with steps outlined elsewhere in this book. It must be stressed, however, that these changes in the SSDI program will benefit only those recipients who want to work. The SSDI rolls include large numbers of individuals who are not interested in resuming employment; these include persons who have retired on disability insurance, widows of disabled persons, and individuals with low employability. For those who do desire to work, however, the changes listed below will be salutary and, together with other recommended improvements, of potentially great importance.[3]

1. *Discount Work-Related Costs from SGA.* The precedent Tom Brown established has yet to be incorporated into SSDI regulations or legislated by amendments to the social-security laws. This proposal would permit persons who require special equipment, transportation, attendant-care services, or other support in order to work to deduct the value or cost of these services from earnings in determining SGA. It would be a major work incentive. And it is equitable, because it would establish for severely disabled persons who need extraordinary investments to work the ability to earn as much "real" income as those who are less disabled and require little or no special services for employment. The cost to the SSDI program of making this change is relatively modest, consisting largely of the minor increase in the number of persons who would become (or remain) eligible for benefits, and most likely would not exceed $5 million per year, or $1 per person benefiting from SSDI at present.

2. *Continue Medicare Eligibility Following Termination from SSDI Rolls.* The sudden loss of all Medicare coverage subsequent to termination is one of the greatest work disincentives in the program. If the cash benefits were to be suspended but Medicare coverage continued, more beneficiaries would take a chance on employment. The costs associated with this option are minor, as only those who actually return to work would be affected. The advantages, however, are major. First, the Medicare coverage is of critical importance in itself for many severely disabled

people. Second, eligibility for Medicare often provides access to state-supported medical coverage as well, thus expanding the benefits. Third, should employment terminate for whatever reason, re-establishment of SSDI eligibility for cash benefits would be much smoother and quicker than it is at present (the fear of two full years without coverage is a huge obstacle to employment for many disabled individuals). Ideally, the continuation of coverage would be as permanent as required by the individual, so that, for example, if his employer did not cover him under a private plan he would still be protected. At a minimum, seven years of continued coverage would be needed in order for the extension of protection to serve as an incentive to return to work. Permanent coverage might be offered in the near future, at any rate, through some kind of national health insurance. While it is difficult to put a price tag on this option, it is unlikely that the costs would exceed $50 million yearly, or $10 per person.

3. Eliminate Two-Year Waiting Period for Medicare. For persons who have already established eligibility for SSDI, and who have left the rolls to go to work (or who have lost cash benefits under the option above and who have worked beyond the Medicare-coverage period), loss of a job should permit immediate reinstatement of Medicare coverage. The cost of removing this two-year waiting period would be approximately $25 million per year. A more expensive proposal (because it might attract more people to SSDI rolls) is elimination of the original two-year waiting period for Medicare eligibility as well. Despite its possible high cost, it is worth considering because of the crucial importance of coverage to severely disabled persons, who cannot afford adequate medical coverage otherwise.

4. Expand the Trial-Work Period and Raise Allowable Earnings. At present, SSDI beneficiaries are allowed a nine-month "trial-work period," during which they may test their ability to engage in "substantial gainful activity." The nine-month period, however, is quite short. Even more serious is the limit upon earnings: $50 earned in a single month is counted as a trial-work month. It is highly doubtful that the capacity to earn $50 a month for nine not necessarily consecutive months establishes an ability to work independently. At a minimum, twenty-four months should be allowed and beneficiaries should be permitted to earn up to SGA (currently $240/month) before a month is counted toward the trial-work total. An additional advantage of extending the trial-work period to twenty-four months is that persons who are clients of vocational rehabilitation agencies would be assured of continued benefits for the duration of the services (which may last as long as eighteen months). Extension of the trial-work period to twenty-four months would cost approximately $10 million per year, or $2 per person benefiting from SSDI at present.

5. Increase Support for Beneficiary Rehabilitation Program (BRP). The 1965 Social Security Amendments created the BRP as part of the SSDI program, offering state rehabilitation agencies 100% reimbursement for costs of all SSDI beneficiaries who were rehabilitated and removed from the rolls, up to a statutory limit (currently 1.5% of the previous year's SSDI payments). The funds are made available to the state agencies quarterly. The purposes of the BRP are to produce savings in the SSDI program by removing persons who can be trained for work from the rolls and to provide persons who can work with the rehabilitation services they need to obtain jobs. The program has proven to be successful, returning significant savings to the SSDI trust fund, although it has also received heavy criticism for not doing enough. In recent years, only 1.5% of all beneficiaries have been rehabilitated and terminated from the rolls. The low rate of termination through rehabilitation is attributable in part to the disincentives to employment inherent in the SSDI program, in part to the fact that employment opportunities for many disabled persons are nonexistent or at least very difficult to locate, and in part to the fact that SSDI rehabilitation monies are exhausted early in each quarter by rehabilitation agencies. Increasing the amount allocated for rehabilitation of beneficiaries (to 2.5% of the previous year's payment level, for example) would offer additional funds but would not of course remove the disincentive or employment obstacles.

6. *Raise the SGA Limit.* At present, all disabled individuals seeking SSDI benefits are limited to the SGA income restriction of $240 per month, or $2,880 per year. Blind individuals, by contrast, are permitted to earn up to the earnings limit for retired persons aged 65–72; in 1978, this limit was $4,000 per year, and it is scheduled to increase to $6,000 annually by 1982. (The social-security system separates "blind" from "disabled" persons.) Thus, persons who are blind may earn $190 per month more than other persons who are disabled before losing eligibility for SSDI. The difference reflects political more than needs factors; blind persons and their advocates historically have been better organized and more powerful than other groups of disabled people. There is no inherent rea-

son for blind persons to benefit from a higher SGA level than that allowed other disabled individuals. The objection might be raised that to increase the SGA limit would entice more people to stay on the rolls. The facts, however, indicate that a higher proportion of blind than nonblind SSDI beneficiaries are now working. There is reason to believe, then, that increasing the SGA to an equitable level, one shared by aged, blind, and disabled persons, would serve as a work incentive for disabled individuals.

The real potential in rehabilitating beneficiaries will occur when changes proposed in other chapters are implemented. With disabled people receiving better education, improved rehabilitation services, facing fewer barriers to mobility, and having more employment opportunities, the numbers on SSDI rolls should drop dramatically.

Medical Dependency Factors[4]

I have already alluded to medical-care costs incurred by disabled persons in the discussion of Medicare protection under SSDI and shall consider them again below with respect to Medicaid coverage under Supplemental Security Income (SSI). These costs can be staggering.

The cost of medical care is three times as great for disabled persons as it is for nondisabled individuals. As a proportion of income, the median cost of such care is five times as great for disabled as for nondisabled individuals. Severely disabled persons are hospitalized four times as often as nondisabled individuals, and for three times as long per stay. Annual per-capita costs of hospital care, physicians' services, and other medical charges for severely disabled persons are, respectively, five times, three times, and twice those of nondisabled persons using similar kinds of services.

It has been estimated that an individual who is para- plegic, that is, unable to control his foot and leg move- ments voluntarily, must earn $12,000 annually just to be able to afford the same kind of medical coverage available from Medicare/Medicaid. A quadriplegic, who has no vol- untary control of arms or legs, must earn $18,000 for the same amount of coverage.[5] Such incomes are rare; most severely disabled people earn considerably less than $3,000 annually. Accordingly, coverage by Medicare or Medicaid becomes crucial. Data from the 1972 Social Secu- rity Survey of Disabled and Nondisabled Adults indicate that while 85% of the U.S. population aged 20–64 had private health insurance coverage, only 58% of severely disabled and 69% of all disabled persons had such cover- age.

The costs to society of health care for disabled individu- als are very large and are increasing at a rate much faster than that of inflation. Berkowitz and Rubin have studied these expenses over the past decade. Their findings are startling. In 1967, medical payments attributable to disabil- ity were $21 billion, of which $8 billion was spent by the federal government, $3 billion by state and local govern- ments, and $10 billion by the private sector. Three years later, in 1970, the medical payments total was $33.5 billion. In that year, the federal share was $13.8 billion, with $4.3 billion spent by state and local governments, and $15.4 billion by the private sector. By 1973, the federal share had increased to $19.9 billion of the $46.6 billion total, with state and local expenditures at $5.9 billion and private spending at $20.8 billion. In 1975, the medical payments total was $65 billion, with $29 billion on the federal level, $6.5 billion on the state and local level, and $29.5 billion in the private sector. Berkowitz and Rubin expect the medical-payments total for 1980 to be approximately $104 billion.

These figures illustrate the spiralling costs of medical care for disabled individuals. Between 1970 and 1975, medical costs increased 95%, largely because of increases in the number of beneficiaries and expanding coverage for these persons. The federal increase was even larger during this period, growing at 110% over just five years. Even after correcting for inflation, medical-cost increases between 1970 and 1975 rose 40%, with the federal share increasing by 52%.

If we look at the proportion of SSDI beneficiaries covered by Medicare, we find it to be better than eight in ten. Almost three million disabled workers, children of beneficiaries, and widows and widowers receive monthly Medicare benefits.

But large numbers of disabled people are not covered by Medicare. Even those who are on the SSDI rolls had to wait twenty-nine months before receiving Medicare coverage: five months after onset of disability to qualify for SSDI and an additional twenty-four months before Medicare coverage began. Almost one out every three beneficiaries had no comprehensive health coverage to protect them during that twenty-nine-month waiting period. And it is precisely here, during the first few months following onset of the disability, that medical-care costs are highest—and the ability of the individual to absorb them lowest.

Resolution of these complex problems depends upon

a number of initiatives. It will be essential for the nation to invest substantial resources in medical research aimed at preventing disability itself and at restoring ability as quickly as possible among those who do become disabled. We do know that early intervention, preferably within one week of onset, can dramatically alleviate the effects of a disability—and the costs associated with it. Some form of national health insurance is expected to be needed if disabled persons are to be covered for their extraordinary medical costs during these critical first months. Other options include broadening employment-related health-insurance policies to include coverage of medical costs following the onset of disability, whether or not the injury was job related. Some employer insurance plans already do offer medical coverage for up to two years following the termination of employment of persons who must leave their jobs because of disability. Another possibility would be to make insurance available for purchase irrespective of the purchaser's disability; the premiums under this option would likely be too high for most disabled individuals, however.

Regardless of the options chosen, two problems are unavoidable. One is the highly inflationary growth of medical-care costs generally; these costs hurt all Americans, but they harm disabled and elderly persons more than most others because of the relatively low incomes of these persons, large proportions of which must go for medical care, and because of the higher-than-normal utilization of medical care by these individuals. Hospital-cost containment, proposed by the Carter administration in 1978 but not enacted at that time, will be of critical importance for disabled and elderly people. And too, the costs associated with health care for disabled and old people must not lead us

to deprive these individuals of adequate care. No society
that really cared about the value of human life would deny
essential services on the basis that costs are "too high."
We must find ways to reduce the costs and to make the
protection more widely available if disabled and elderly
people are to become more independent and self-sufficient.

SSI: Guaranteeing a Minimum Income

The Supplemental Security Income (SSI) program differs
in several important respects from the SSDI program.
While the latter is available for persons who have demonstrated a capacity to work, the former is open to poor
disabled individuals who may never have worked. And
while SSDI is primarily an insurance program designed
to protect workers who become disabled, SSI is an income-
maintenance program provided to ensure that eligible persons, including poor elderly and disabled individuals, have
a certain minimum income level.

The 1972 amendments to the social-security act combined programs for elderly, blind, and disabled persons
into a new Title XVI, the Supplemental Security Income
Program. The program attempts to provide a minimum-
income base for individuals who are unable to support
themselves because of age, blindness, or disability and who
have limited resources to draw upon to meet the costs
of living.

Disability is defined by reference to "substantial gainful
activity," or SGA: the applicant must be "unable to engage
in any substantial gainful activity by reason of any medically
determinable physical or mental impairment which can be

expected to result in death or which has lasted or can be expected to last for a continuous period of not less than 12 months." Usually, medical documentation by a physician suffices to establish disability. SGA is set, as in SSDI, at $240 per month.

The intent of the program is to ensure that recipients will have a minimum monthly income of $189.40. Thus, SSI funds supplement other income to the extent that this other income falls below the minimum level. Take, for example, the case of a man earning $200 per month and receiving $100 monthly from an annuity. To determine eligibility for SSI, the earned income is subjected to an initial exclusion of $65 per month, with the balance halved. Thus, $200 minus $65 is $135, half of which is $67.50. This is his "countable earned income." Twenty dollars of unearned income is also discountable, so $80 of the annuity is countable unearned income. The total of earned and unearned income is $147.50. The SSI monthly payment then will be $41.90, or the difference between $147.50 and the guaranteed minimum of $189.40.

Why would an individual seek SSI eligibility for such a modest monthly payment? The answer, as in SSDI, relates to the benefits and services which are contingent upon SSI eligibility. State supplemental payments, for example, are often available. Referral to vocational rehabilitation agencies for evaluation and, if appropriate, training is required for all SSI applicants. Children who are eligible for SSI may be referred to a state agency providing services to disabled children. SSI eligibility also enables recipients to benefit from the Agriculture Department's food-stamp program. Beneficiaries are eligible for Title XX social-service programs, which offer a wide array of assistance: day care, consumer education, counseling, foster care, health services, home-delivered meals, housing-improvement services, legal assistance, training, and transportation services. SSI eligibility also qualifies a disabled person for Housing and Urban Development (HUD) "Section 8" rent subsidies. The recipient pays between 15% and 25% of his or her income for rent and HUD picks up the difference between this amount and the monthly rent that would be charged on the open market.

For many disabled individuals, however, the most important service made available through SSI eligibility is Medicaid. States qualifying for federal matching funds under this program are required to provide certain services to disabled SSI recipients, including physician services, inpatient and outpatient hospital services, transportation to and from medical-service facilities, and screening and diagnostic services. States may also offer prosthetic services, private nursing, physical therapy, and other home health services to SSI recipients. For children, the EPSDT (Early and Periodic Screening, Diagnosis and Treatment Program) services made available as part of the SSI program may assist in prompt identification of disability and regular physician care for illnesses and impairments.

The two million SSI beneficiaries who are disabled differ markedly from SSDI recipients. Generally, those eligible for SSI are younger and less well educated. More of them are women and more are members of racial and ethnic minorities. SSI recipients who are disabled usually became disabled earlier in life and have been disabled for a longer period of time than is the case with SSDI beneficiaries. Compared with SSDI-eligible persons, they had less-skilled jobs, earned less, and had participated less in the labor market. For all of these reasons, few SSI recipients can qualify for SSDI.

The "substantial gainful activity" (SGA) limit on earnings is even more devastating upon SSI applicants and recipients than is the case with SSDI because the SGA limit is imposed as a second restriction upon income over the regular SSI income determination. That is, an individual must first be determined to be "poor" according to SSI regulations, and then to be "poorer" under the SGA test. Thus, while $65 of earnings and 50% of the remaining earned income is disregarded for the purpose of establishing eligibility—in an effort to encourage persons to work—the SGA limit establishes a ceiling on such earnings, thus effectively working at cross-purposes with the rest of the program. We should not be surprised, then, to find that fewer than 4% of SSI recipients report any earned income.

The work-disincentive effect of defining employment that pays half the minimum wage as "substantial" and of restricting income to no more than two-thirds of the official poverty level can be readily appreciated. To illustrate this effect, consider the story of Lynn Thompson.

LYNN THOMPSON: A CASE HISTORY[6]

Lynn Thompson was twenty-seven when she killed herself on February 6, 1978. "I don't want you to think of this as suicide," she said in a tape recording left for her family. "Think of it as R&R forever."

Lynn had worked for three years as a night dispatcher for Olsten's Health Care Services of Los Angeles. She did the work at home in her apartment, because muscular dystrophy kept her from seeking employment elsewhere. Out of her earnings, as much as $492 per month, she paid her rent and other expenses. Her SSI eligibility permitted her to qualify for MediCal (California's medical insurance program), including a live-in personal-care attendant, whose services she needed for dressing, eating, and other daily activities.

Two months before her suicide, Lynn received a letter from the Social Security Administration telling her that because she had exceeded SGA limits on earnings, she was no longer eligible for SSI benefits. The letter indicated that her payments, health coverage, and other services were being terminated, and ordered her to pay back $10,000 in past benefits.

Lynn quickly calculated that she would no longer be able to survive. Her rent was only $11 per month less than her $390 SSI benefits (she needed an apartment large enough to accommodate the attendant as well as herself). On the tape, she explained why she could not go on:

"Anyway, I need a rest. . . . This has got to be too much of a hassle, the whole thing. It's just a matter of time before the county catches up with me anyway so they'll cut me off too. Then I *would* be in trouble . . . without the attendant money.

"No one's to blame. I mean, it's my own doing, you know? You wanna call it a cop-out or a chicken-out or whatever, you know, that's fine. I just didn't feel like going through this hassle any more.

"Don't worry. Everything's cool. I just want all of you to know that I'll miss you, I love you very much, I couldn't ask for a better family or friends, even if I could have selected them myself. So, I love you all very much. . . .

". . . I have a couple more requests. First, there's no

need for a big hullabaloo. Just plant me and get it over
with. And, secondly, give the Social Security Office a message for me. Tell them thanks for being the straw that
broke the camel's back.

"I realize the system's here to help people but it needs
some going over. It'd be great if I could work or support
myself and still receive the full attendant benefits and, of
course, some kind of medical benefits. But the county has
the same margins. Anything over $296 is considered extra
money. Therefore, anything I make over $296, that's how
much I can be shortened in the months to follow. So it
makes no difference if I'm working 15 hours a day, Monday
through Friday, 8 hours a day Saturday and Sunday, or
if I worked an extra day or if I worked holidays to make
extra pay. It doesn't make any difference. They're still going to cut me off that much more, you know. So, really,
you're working for nothing."

Her supervisor said Lynn was a "spectacular human being, a source of inspiration to everybody who had anything
to do with her—a young woman who in essence was totally
self-sufficient, but who had a degenerating disease so every
day was a little worse than the day before."

One month later, on March 1, the State of California
put into effect a law passed the year before that permitted
severely disabled persons to earn larger amounts while
retaining attendant-care and other MediCal benefits. But
it was too late for Lynn Thompson.

Reforming SSI

1. Raise the SGA Limit. Increasing SGA from $240 to
$800 per month for all recipients is relatively inexpensive

yet would permit many more disabled and elderly persons who need medical, education, day-care, and other services to receive this assistance. It would also provide a more realistic test of the ability to work prior to suspension of benefits at termination. The cost would be approximately $15 million annually, or the equivalent of $7 per year per person for every disabled person now on SSI.

2. *Discount Work-Related Expenses.* This proposal, similar in concept to its counterpart in SSDI, would be relatively inexpensive but equitable, helping severely disabled persons reach more of a par with less severely disabled individuals with respect to "real" allowable earnings. At present, a disabled person may deduct from his or her earnings only expenses connected solely with work and only those which nondisabled workers do not incur.

3. *Continue Medicaid Coverage.* The arguments for this proposal parallel those made earlier with respect to Medicare under SSDI. Note, however, that there is no Medicaid waiting period under SSI.

These three proposals would create work incentives for many SSI recipients. Because all earned income above $65 per month is computed in determining monthly payments, the more recipients earn themselves the less SSI must pay. In fact, if only 12% of the recipients were to seek and obtain work paying less than the proposed SGA level, the savings to the program would be about $2,000 per person per year, or $150 million to $200 million annually.

Bridging the Gap

The reform proposals presented in this chapter are modest in nature. They will not by themselves dramatically curtail the costs associated with dependence among disabled and elderly people, although they will contribute markedly to halting the growth that has characterized these costs over the past decade. The importance of the changes is that, in conjunction with improvements in employment training and opportunities, these reforms will bridge the gap between the present system, in which dependence costs threaten the stability of our economy, and the possible future, in which millions of disabled and elderly persons turn from being tax-users to becoming tax-payers.

That the gap will not be bridged without such changes is readily apparent. Despite the fact that referrals to vocational-rehabilitation agencies are mandatory for all SSDI and SSI recipients, only a very small proportion of these recipients are rehabilitated to employment. The threat of losing Medicare or Medicaid coverage, which is worth between $2,000 and $5,000 annually for most disabled persons, is a serious disincentive. Similarly, the current SGA levels do not permit a disabled individual sufficient time to determine if he or she is capable of supporting himself or herself. And the economy does not now offer jobs for undereducated, undertrained, and severely disabled and elderly individuals that are sufficiently stable and well paying to enable these individuals to leave benefit rolls with confidence.

The Tom Browns and Lynn Thompsons among us want to work. They believe that with the necessary supportive services they can become self-sufficient, independent citizens. What these proposals aim to accomplish is to offer them an opportunity to move from dependence to independence. And if that does not exemplify the very core of the American dream, I do not know what does.

Meeting the Challenge:
Dependence Reform

This will be the least expensive of the five steps, yet the others cannot go forward to any appreciable extent without it. We must eliminate the disincentives that discourage people from seeking improved education, rehabilitation, and employment, and, at the same time, we must encourage people to avoid dependence rolls whenever possible. Combined with the other steps proposed in this book, the investments we make in dependence reform will pay for themselves many times over as people leave the rolls and enter payrolls.

As part of the ten-year, $22-billion-a-year plan, I am proposing that we spend a total of $2.2-billion on the four levels. The bulk of this spending will be on the federal level, especially if some form of national health insurance is enacted and if welfare becomes more federalized. While private spending will be minimal, benefits should be large as the individual and corporate income taxes, social-security taxes, and other expenditures are cut. Although the continued rapid increase in the aging population may prevent an actual cut in these taxes or a rebate, the reductions in disability expenditures will at least slow any increase in overall spending and taxation.

In making the calculations, I took into account the fact that advances in education, rehabilitation, barrier removal, and other parts of the plan would make it possible for many people to become less dependent on social-security and other rolls within five or six years. Accordingly, I am suggesting a gradual increase in spending to 1984, with a sharp decline thereafter. Specifically, the amounts I suggest are $250 million in 1981, $350 million in 1982–84, $300 million in 1985, $250 million in 1986, $150 million in 1987, $100 million in 1988, and $50 million in 1989–90. The amounts would continue to decline, but gradually, because some persons would not be able to leave the rolls permanently and may re-enter or remain in the system.

6 The Open Community

As you look around your own community, you will doubtless see innumerable examples of how America handicaps disabled and elderly people. You will see physical barriers, such as steep flights of stairs, communication barriers, such as audio announcements in stores and transportation terminals that deaf people cannot hear, and attitudinal barriers, such as a neighborhood's refusal to permit the opening of a hostel for retarded youth. Considering these, knowing that similar obstacles appear in virtually every American city and county, and understanding that *you* are paying for these barriers through unnecessarily high income, social-security, and other taxes, you may become disturbed that the barriers are not being removed. And as you think about these problems, you may wonder why those barriers are there at all.

America has handicapped disabled people and elderly citizens for two hundred years. Every citizen is now paying for this tragic miscarriage of justice. But disabled and elderly people have been paying for two centuries. Those of us who are disabled and those who are old want to join those of you who are "temporarily able-bodied" in a partnership to remove the barriers that cost all of us too much. We want to work together to create a barrier-free America.

What is it that you, an average citizen, can do? This thought may have occurred to you repeatedly in previous chapters. Not all of us can do research, design buildings, build buses, teach disabled children, or do rehabilitation counseling, nor can all of us mount political pressure powerful enough to influence federal and state legislation. But there is much that each of us can accomplish, vitally important tasks both small and large that will do as much as anything to help disabled and elderly people, and America itself.

Identifying Barriers

The first step in any community is to discover precisely what it is that presents obstacles to disabled and elderly persons. Barriers are readily recognized, once you know what to look for. What must be done depends upon what the barriers are, where they are, and who is responsible for their removal.

What exactly is a "barrier?" Let's look at three broad categories of barriers and then examine each more carefully.

Societal Barriers. Lack of knowledge about and understanding of disability and age is a major barrier. It can be removed through a wide variety of educational approaches. Steps you can take include asking television and radio stations in your area to interview disabled or elderly adults who live in the community, asking your newspaper to run a series of articles by a local expert on disability, asking the school board to require some instruction on disability at all levels of the school system, and asking community associations such as Rotary Clubs, Lions Clubs, Chambers of Commerce, Jaycees, and churches to feature disability- and age-related issues in their programs.

Stereotyping is a closely related barrier. You can help to remove it by offering people who hold stereotyped beliefs information which challenges their beliefs. Stereotypes usually arise from a concentration, not on a person's abilities, but on disability or age. Thus, introducing a successful disabled adult, sharing books written by or about disabled or old people and their work, and other approaches can be very helpful. Perhaps no approach is quite so dramatic as is role reversal and simulation training. You could host a "street fair" at which people can use wheelchairs, hearing aids and other devices, and talk with disabled people. When someone sits in a chair and is asked if he or she is less of a human being for that fact, and when he or she learns from a paraplegic individual how to manipulate the chair and do "impossible things" with it, stereotypes begin to fall.[7]

Requirements pose yet another societal barrier. Many of these bear no factual relationship to the activity they regulate. The next time you apply for a job, for example, study the job description closely. Is it actually necessary for a secretary to "hear a whisper from across a room" or for a teacher to be able to see perfectly?

Architectural Barriers. The most obvious of all barriers, these may be costly to remove, and you may have to be accordingly persistent and ingenious to succeed. In addition to *steps* where no elevators exist, architectural barriers include *doors* that revolve or that are narrower than thirty-two inches, *elevators* that have controls too high to reach from a wheelchair or that are too small to permit a chair to enter and turn around, *corridors* that are less than five feet across, *drinking fountains* and *telephones* that are too high to reach, *bus floors* that are not accompanied by ramps or lifts, and *parking spaces* that do not have sufficient space to enable a person to place a wheelchair beside the car to exit and enter.

You can help remove architectural barriers in a number of ways. If the facility is a private business, you may alert the owner to the barrier, cite statistics on the number of disabled and old people who cannot enter to purchase his products, cite the Tax Reform Act provision allowing up to $25,000 in tax deductions for alterations, and appeal to his public image in the community. If all of this does not work, you can talk with the local business association to which he belongs or to other civic-minded groups to see what they can do. If this fails, you can talk with some disabled and elderly persons to see if they would like to visit the owner or even stage a "media event" in which the press would accompany them in their attempt to enter the facility.

If the facility benefits from federal financial assistance, as most schools, libraries, colleges, hospitals, and social-service programs do, you have more options. You may file a complaint with the Department of Health, Education, and Welfare in Washington, D.C., telling the agency the exact nature of the problem, when you discovered it, and (to the extent you know this) who if anyone has been discriminated against because of the problem, together with your name and address. You, or a disabled person who has been discriminated against, may also go to court. The law (P.L. 95–602) provides that attorneys' fees will be paid by the government if the court action is successful, while if it is not, the lawyer usually will not expect to be paid.[8]

If the facility is a federally owned or leased building, you can file a complaint with the Architectural and Transportation Barrier Compliance Board in Washington, D.C. The board's staff will investigate.

If the company or organization which uses the facility has contracts with the federal government, as most large companies do, you can write to the Department of Labor in Washington, D.C. New regulations provide that contractors must make at least one entrance to the facility, the hiring or personnel office, and selected worksites fully accessible.

If progress in any of these areas is slow, you will have to do a little more. Ask a local organization of disabled or elderly people if it would hold a press conference charging that the facility is inaccessible. Particularly where federal funds are involved, this may get good results: the ultimate penalty for violations is termination of all government money and debarment from future government business. This will affect, not only disabled and elderly people, but everyone who uses the facility, so the press should be interested.

Other steps you can take include organizing a boycott of a store or company, writing letters to the editor of the local papers, or even demonstrating in the street in front of the facility.

Communication Barriers. These may include stores, hotels, and other buildings and facilities used by the public that have flashing-light alarms but *no auditory alarms* for fire or other emergencies, no provision for warning deaf people of impending events (in a hotel, for example, it is rare for a light to be installed in the room to alert the deaf person that someone is calling on him or that his phone is ringing and a message is being taken for him; in a bus terminal, train station, or airport, it may mean auditory but not visual announcements of arrivals and de-partures), *essential services provided in one medium but not in another* (examples include printed but not brailled menus, spoken but not interpreted speeches or lectures, "walk/ wait" signals which do not have buzzers, and similar prob-lems), *entertainment offered that only some people can benefit from* (e.g., uncaptioned movies and television, lack of brailled or recorded summaries of settings and scenes for blind theatregoers, et cetera), and *safety devices that screen people out* (e.g., apartment lobby telephones that deaf people can-not use, elevator phones, et cetera). Other communication barriers include *sales clerks and other public service personel who do not know how to assist deaf and blind persons* to make purchases, place telephone calls, and secure information.

Often, it will be sufficient to alert the manager or owner to the problem and offer a resource from which the neces-sary devices or training may be secured. (A resource guide is provided later in this chapter.) For pervasive problems, consider asking church groups or other civic-minded asso-ciations to take on as one of their projects the removal of communication barriers in the community.

Organizing for Action

Effecting change on the local, state, and national level is difficult for individual citizens to accomplish but much easier for groups. Most effective are "coalitions" of groups, which consist of a number of organizations and associations pooling resources to work on problems of common concern. You are most likely to be able to forge coalitions by contacting groups which are "natural allies" of disabled and elderly people. These include parent associations, labor unions, churches, civil-rights organizations, and business groups. A coalition gives you two things you really need in order to bring pressure to bear upon your target, who is of course the person(s) who can remove the barrier. First, coalitions provide large numbers of people who care about the issue and are prepared to do something about it. The more people you represent the more effective you can be. Second, coalitions permit efficient use of limited resources. Public-relations and political campaigns can be time consuming and expensive. By joining together, you make it possible for one group to supply postage and envelopes, another to gather volunteers, a third to visit media officials, a fourth to secure expert assistance from specialists in barrier removal, and so forth. Remember that politicians are accountable to voters, school boards to parents and members of the community, businessmen to customers. The more of the right people you represent, the more likely your target will listen to you—and act.

The targets in this case are mayors and city-council members, local educators, private businessmen, state assemblymen, governors, agency heads, senators and congressmen, and the president of the United States. Sometimes, as when residents of a community, acting out of fear and ignorance, protest the placement in the community of retarded individuals, another group must act out of courage and understanding to support the hostel. At other times, media officials who are perpetuating stereotypes of disabled and elderly people must be confronted with the facts. Your coalition has to be flexible, know its goals, find its targets, and act in a timely and effective fashion.

Are you concerned about the federal government's unremitting opposition to funding the state-federal rehabilitation program? Then send letters, very early in the summer, to the president and the secretary of Health, Education, and Welfare. Present the facts as you see them, then explain why you are willing to act on this issue. Tell them what spending on rehabilitation means to you in terms of your taxes and other problems you face. Do large companies in your community discriminate against disabled and elderly people? If so, organize your activities on both the local and the national level. Locally, you will want to generate public-relations, consumer, and other kinds of pressure; nationally, you will want to be sure that the Department of Labor investigates the issue and takes whatever action might be appropriate.

Does your governor oppose increasing support for state and local education for disabled children? If so, concentrate upon generating pressure on him or her from the state assembly, "natural allies" of disabled people such as unions and parent groups, and voters throughout the state. Media exposure may be especially effective. Are local restaurants, theatres, sports centers, recreational programs, museums, and other entertainment and leisure activities closed to disabled and elderly people? Consider the full range of options open to your coalition—meeting with the owners and managers, press coverage, boycotts, demonstrations, and others, including protests to the Department of Health, Education, and Welfare if section 504 is involved.

Is there no public transportation available for disabled and elderly people in your community? Consider meeting with the mayor, the city council, the transportation authority, and other officials. A mass walkout (refusal to use public transit on a given day) is another possibility. Working for a referendum or petition for purchase of the Transbus, the fully accessible mass-transit vehicle, is yet another.

In all of your work, be sure you have possession of the facts. Take advantage of resources of assistance and information. Some are listed below.

Where to Get Help

While barriers are relatively simple to identify, knowing how to remove them inexpensively is more difficult. Fortunately, there are numerous sources from which you can obtain free information and technical assistance. The first and most important is the disabled and elderly population of the community itself. If you do not know how to find these groups, write a letter to the American Coalition of Citizens with Disabilities, Inc., Washington, D.C. 20005. The coalition maintains regular contact with more than three thousand such groups nationwide.

For information and assistance on barrier removal, contact:

The National Center for a Barrier-Free Environment
Gallaudet College
Seventh and Florida, N.E.
Washington, D.C. 20002

Architectural and Transportation Barriers Compliance Board
Washington, D.C. 20201

American Institute of Architects
1735 New York Avenue, N.W.
Washington, D.C. 20006

Some publications that might help you include:

American National Standards Institute (ANSI) Specification for Making Buildings and Facilities Accessible to and Usable by the Physically Handicapped. New York: Author, 1961 and revised edition. Write to: ANSI, 1430 Broadway, New York, New York 10018. This is the standard reference work in the area.

Accessibility Assistance: A Directory of Consultants on Environments for Handicapped People. Washington, D.C.: National Center for a Barrier-Free Environment, 1978. (Address above.) Lists engineers, architects, designers, planners, and communication-barrier specialists nationwide, including those who provide services and information free of charge.

Opening Doors: A Guide to Making Facilities Accessible to Handicapped People. Washington, D.C.: National Center for a Barrier-Free Environment, 1978. Offers a simple, yet accurate, guide to accessible design.

The latter two publications were produced with support from the Community Services Administration, the federal antipoverty agency. CSA also offers several very helpful publications on how to influence policy-making in the community and in the federal government. Especially helpful is *Citizen Participation* (1978). For your copy, write to CSA, 1200 Nineteenth Street, N.W., Washington, D.C. 20506. A series of "citizen-action guides" is published by the Center for Community Change, 1000 Wisconsin Avenue, N.W., Washington, D.C. 20007. Two of the best are:

Citizen Involvement in Community Development: An Opportunity and a Challenge (1978)

Citizen Involvement in the Budget Process (1978)

The Center for Governmental Studies, P.O. Box 34481, Washington, D.C. 20034, offers a monthly bulletin and a series of articles on citizen involvement in local budgeting, planning, and other matters. Tremendously helpful for advocates is a publication of the Coordinating Council for Handicapped Children in Chicago called *How to Organize an Effective Parent Group and Move Bureaucracies*. Published in 1971, it may be out of print, so I suggest you contact a local public-school library or teacher's college for a copy. The American Coalition of Citizens with Disabilities publishes two books you may want: *Coalition Building* (1978) and *Planning Effective Advocacy Programs* (1979). For copies, write to ACCD, Washington, D.C. 20005.

The Last Barrier

If America handicaps disabled and elderly people, it is because all of us have made it so. In the end, it is not just the physical, communication, and attitudinal barriers that disabled and elderly people confront that handicap them and America: it is also the beliefs and actions of these persons themselves. Those of us who are disabled or old have to go through many of the same stages blacks and women went through before us. We must come to value ourselves, set our goals high, and determine that we will overcome whatever barriers we find.

Disabled and elderly people are not responsible for being handicapped, but they are responsible for becoming rehabilitated. It is not their fault the barriers exist, but it is their fault if they do not surmount them. To adopt Jesse Jackson's words, they are not responsible for being down, but they are responsible for getting up.

Bringing It All Together

I have outlined in this chapter some steps for rehabilitating America by working in the community. It will require your direct and personal involvement to succeed. Why should you implement this plan, or some version of it? I can think of two compelling reasons. First, it will more than pay for itself; that is, we as a country will benefit, today. And second, it will help us create an affordable future.

A Better Present. Inflation, poverty, big government, and increased longevity are imposing unnecessarily heavy burdens upon us. Our income, social-security, state, and local taxes are higher than they need to be. When we can attack these problems, and at a negative cost, we should do it. The removal of barriers will enable all of us to move about with more ease and safety. Accidents will be cut, deaths prevented. Our growing economy needs all the human and financial resources at our command. We cannot afford to ignore the contributions of thirty-six million disabled persons and twenty-five million elderly citizens. And the research and technology innovations designed to assist disabled people will produce spin-offs that will help all of us.

An Affordable Future. The uncontrollable segment of the federal budget is three-fourths of all federal expenditures. Some of this is genuinely uncontrollable, but much is not, especially spending on dependence among disabled and elderly persons. The rate at which this spending is increasing will result in its doubling in size within eight years if we do not move to halt and reverse it. The sooner we move, the less costly will be the effort and the greater the return. Consider, for example, spending on elderly persons between 1969 and 1979. During this ten-year period, allocations rose from $40 billion to $153 billion and from one-fifth of the federal budget to one-third. The impact upon our income taxes and social-security taxes has been devastating. We face an even more disastrous situation in the next ten years if we do not act now.

In February 1979, the Washington *Post* ran a front-page story by Peter Milius entitled, "Social Security: Some Good News." Milius reported that the number of persons qualifying for disability insurance under the Social Security Disability Insurance program had declined in recent years to the 1972 level. The decline, still modest in size, was enough, he said, to spur many in Congress to consider rescinding the just enacted social-security tax increases. One-third of that increase had been required to meet anticipated disability-insurance costs. The decline, then, meant that the program was now operating with a surplus, making a cut of two or three hundred dollars in every covered worker's tax possible. Accelerating the decline through steps such as those proposed in this book may generate even larger cuts in individual and corporate taxes. This is one aspect of the affordable future.

Another is the fact that persons aged sixty-five now can expect to live an average of sixteen additional years, and the trend toward greater longevity is expected to continue strongly. This means two things with respect to the future of all of us. First, it means that if old people are maintained on dependence programs, the costs will accelerate greatly. The "senior boom" will produce many more senior citizens at the same time as the nation's lowered fertility rate is producing fewer working-age individuals. The result will be a larger burden on each covered worker. The more important second implication of the greater longevity of elderly persons is that the "young old" increasingly are healthy and not only able to work, but frequently willing to do so. Many who do not want to work do wish to contribute meaningfully to the community. If we can rehabilitate these people to employability or productivity, we can generate new resources for our nation while at the same time reducing the burden of dependency upon our taxes. This, too, will help make our future more affordable.

A third aspect is the simple fact that any one of us may at any point "join" the disabled population. The changes we make to benefit disabled people may help each of us tomorrow. Because disability has a devastating effect upon income and standard of living when barriers and other obstacles prevent continued high-level employment, rehabilitating America will help those of us who become disabled live a more affordable future.

Fourth, medical costs are rising out of control. By removing community obstacles, we can help many sick people return home more quickly than they now can, cutting hospital costs. This will be particularly true with respect to elderly persons who are placed in nursing homes but who could live at home if barriers were removed. Equally dramatic in its impact upon medical costs will be prevention and cure of disability. Dependence is recognized as a major cause of both physical and mental illness; by helping people become self-sufficient and independent, we can cut the costs of these illnesses by preventing them. Poverty, too, produces unusually high rates of medical-care usage. The steps proposed in this book will help reduce poverty and thereby the medical expenses it causes. This is yet another aspect of the affordable future.

Finally, we must address the less tangible but even more critical question of affordability in terms not just of costs but also of the quality of life. There can be no question that the standard of living of disabled and elderly people can be improved greatly when a strategy such as proposed here is followed. Huge as the impact of research, barrier removal, education and rehabilitation, and dependence-system reform will be, perhaps the most meaningful contribution will be made by the efforts of those in the disabled or elderly person's neighborhood and community to make him or her feel a valued member of the population, a person seen not so much as someone who can't as someone who can. True equality will never arrive for disabled or old people until this step is taken. And by taking it, we enrich our own lives as well because we are affirming our own humanity and living up to the highest ideals upon which our nation was founded. The future that disabled and elderly people, and the rest of us, will enjoy will be more affordable, then, not only in the economic sense, but also in the psychological sense. For we can afford not just to exist but to live.

Meeting the Challenge: The Open Community

Placing a dollar figure on the final of the five steps is more difficult than it is in other areas, in part because so many of the components of this stage are intangible and in part because there are so many communities in our nation. It is with some trepidation, then, that I make these proposals.

In calculating these costs, I have placed very rough figures on such efforts as community-awareness education programs, revision of unnecessary descriptions of jobs and other requirements for participation in programs and activities, citizen participation in government on behalf of disabled and elderly people, community organizing, and similar activities. Attempting to predict the range of expenditures over ten years was at least as difficult. Finally, assigning the expense to different sectors of society proved somewhat elusive, although clearly much of the expense will be in the private sector. Grants are available from the federal, state, local, and private sectors to finance community efforts, so there will be some impact on all levels.

As part of the ten-year, five-step $22-billion-a-year plan, I am proposing new spending of $12 billion over the coming decade. The costs will rise until about 1984 and then decline gradually as many of the activities reach their goals. In fact, I do not project any additional spending in 1990. Specifically, I estimate that $500 million will be needed in 1981, $1.5 billion in 1982, $2 billion in 1983, $2.5 billion in 1984, $2 billion in 1985, $1.5 billion in 1986, $1 billion in 1987, $750 million in 1988, and $250 million in 1989.

I believe these expenditures will be remarkably effective. We must remember that it is in the community that the person who is disabled or old faces his or her life every day. It is here that he or she finds acceptance and happiness, or they are not found at all. And community action is as traditional as anything in American life. We cannot, nor should we, look only to government for the initiative to solve our problems. The unique thing about community action is that it offers each of us a chance to "do something important" about a problem that concerns us. Working for an open community will help us solve not just one but five problems: inflation, poverty, big government, the burdens of longevity, and disability. And by taking these steps, we are creating a better present and an affordable future for ourselves as well. Few activities are so rewarding, and few are so urgently important. We must become part of the solution of the problem of disability—and we must do it now.

Notes

Preface

1. On inflation and disability, see especially the work of Berkowitz and his colleagues at Rutgers University. I found the mimeographed paper "The Costs of Disability: Estimates of Program Expenditures for Disability, 1967–1975" particularly helpful. Write: Bureau of Economic Research, Rutgers University, New Brunswick, New Jersey 08903. Berkowitz, Johnson, & Murphy (1976) was also useful. Other sources I found invaluable included a speech by HEW Secretary Joseph Califano before the Economic Club of Chicago, April 20, 1978 (for a copy, write to HEW, 200 Independence Avenue, S.W., Washington, D.C. 20201); a *National Journal* article by Robert Samuelson called "Busting the U.S. Budget—The Costs of an Aging America" (1978); another *Journal* story by Robert Hudson (1978); and an Associated Press wire report by Evans Witt (1977).
2. On poverty and disability, see Burdette & Frohlich (1977), Krute & Burdette (1978), Franklin (1977), and Frohlich & Schechter (1977). These reports, by members of the SSA's Division of Disability Studies in the Social Surveys Branch, analyze results of the 1972 SSA survey of disabled and nondisabled adults. For reports on more recent studies (not

available at the time this was written), contact SSA's Office of Research and Statistics, Room 1120, 1875 Connecticut Avenue, N.W., Washington, D.C. 20009. See also Berkowitz, Johnson, & Murphy (1976).

3. The best source of information on the contribution of disability programs to the U.S. budget is, of course, the budget itself. You may obtain a copy of *The Budget of the United States Government, 1980* from the U.S. Government Printing Office, Washington, D.C. 20402. GPO also has available a number of analyses of the budget. Also very helpful is "FY 1980 HEW Budget," available from the department. An analysis of some recent trends may be found in Milius (1979). HEW Secretary Califano said in his Chicago speech that disability insurance, which accounted for $15 billion of HEW's budget in 1980, would require $27 billion just five years later. Trying to give his audience a feeling for the magnitude of these numbers, he noted: "In fact, the one-year increase of $1.4 billion in Social Security disability expenditures from 1977 to 1978—from $11.9 billion to $13.3 billion—will be greater than this year's entire budget of the City of Chicago."

4. On aging and disability, the articles by Samuelson and Hudson are excellent analyses. Some other figures are found in Cohen (1978), who discusses the 1977 social-security amendments at length.

5. The "piece of the pie" quote is Leslie Milk's.

6. Menachem Begin, personal conversation, December 17, 1978. Begin told me he gave some of his prize for scholarships and the bulk for retarded persons. Mrs. Begin heads an Israeli committee on retardation and has contributed greatly to improving the status of retarded people in Israel.

Chapter 1. The Paradox of Costs

1. On the "Me Generation," see in particular Daniel Yankelovich's excellent chapter in the book, *Work in America: The Decade Ahead* (1978), edited by Kerr and Rosow. He refers to the attitudes of modern workers as "New Breed values."

He stresses the fact that paid workers tend not to be motivated toward hard work and instead find their primary rewards in leisure activities.

2. Berkowitz & Rubin (1977) refer to "transfer and medical" programs as opposed to "service" programs. In interpreting their data, I have found it helpful to substitute the terms "dependence" and "independence" for these because what they call transfer and medical expenses are for the most part expenditures on people because they are dependent or because they "can't," while service payments are intended to help people prepare for and perform jobs, thus becoming independent. Berkowitz and Rubin include under "transfer and medical" payments spending on Supplemental Security Income, disability insurance, workmen's compensation, disabled-veterans' benefits, and private insurance benefits, but exclude tax expenditures and survivor's benefits payable to disabled persons. They do not attempt to separate out payments to short- and long-term disabled. Under "service" payments, they include vocational rehabilitation, special education, barrier removal, and "the array of social services that are made available to public assistance recipients," notably Title XX expenditures. Berkowitz and Rubin stress two points. First, high as the costs they find are, "it must be emphasized that we are not talking about the total costs of disability. Those persons who are unable to perform their usual social and work roles have lost a great deal in personal satisfaction and the economy has lost a great deal in terms of the contributions of their productive activity to the welfare of all. These are the significant costs" (pp. 4–5). And second, "there are only three ways to travel. One is to prevent disability from occurring, the second is to control programs by changing eligibility criteria or benefit levels, and the third is to rehabilitate persons so that they can return to productive activity" (p. 5). Berkowitz and Rubin include barrier-removal and civil-rights protection efforts as part of prevention.

3. On labor-force participation by disabled persons, see Bur-

dette & Frohlich (1977) and Krute & Burdette (1978). Also helpful are data from the United States Census, 1970. For an analysis of census data on disability, contact the President's Committee on Employment of the Handicapped, 1111 20th Street, N.W., Washington, D.C. 20036.

4. Franklin (1977) discusses the impact of disability on the family.

5. That rehabilitation agencies can serve only one out of every eleven eligible persons emerged in Congressional hearings prior to the enactment of P.L. 95–602. See *Hearings before the Subcommittee on Select Education of the Committee on Education and Labor, U.S. House of Representatives, January 5, April 7, 10, 11, and 12, 1978.* The 1246-page document, an excellent overview of the state of rehabilitation in 1978, is available from the U.S. Government Printing Office.

6. Burdette & Frohlich (1977) compare 1965 and 1971 labor-force participation and income-maintenance enrollment.

7. Unklesbay's comment was quoted in McCormack (1977).

8. For more information on the Yankelovich survey, contact Yankelovich, Skelly, and White, 575 Madison Avenue, New York, New York. The firm is conducting a follow-up survey at the time of this writing.

9. The 1972 Supreme Court decision on *Papachristou v. City of Jacksonville,* 405, U.S. 156, 164 is the source of the "independence and self-confidence" quote.

Chapter 2. Uncommon Sense

1. George Morris Piersol was quoted by Howard Rusk in congressional testimony before the House Subcommittee on Select Education, April 10, 1978.

2. For data on spending on research related to disability, see especially the report of the Panel on Research Programs to Aid the Handicapped, Committee on Science and Technology, U.S. House of Representatives. Washington, D.C.: U.S. Government Printing Office, 1978.

3. Information on the scientific and technological investiga-

tions discussed in this section may be found in Nicholson (1978), Pines (1978), *Rehabilitation Engineering: A Plan for Continued Progress, II;* Freebairn (1976); *Hearings before the Committee on Science and Technology, Report No. 104, September 22–23, 1976;* Freiberger et al. (1977); and Dudek et al. (1977). Pines is particularly readable. See also her 1973 book, *The Brain Changers* (New York: Harcourt Brace Jovanovich). Boothroyd (1975) discusses technology assisting deaf people, as does Freebairn. An unpublished report by Richard Leclair and Mark Bressler entitled "Compendium of Estimates of Disability and Rehabilitation Device Use" is available from the senior author, Rehabilitation Services Administration, Washington, D.C. 20201. A paper presented by Raymond Kurzweil at the annual meeting of the American Association for the Advancement of Science in 1976, "The Kurzweil Reading Machine—A Technical Overview," is a fascinating account of the struggle to develop the first prototype of this machine. It illustrates the problems facing science and technology in moving machines from prototypes to mass production more vividly than any other paper I have seen. For a copy, write to AAAS, 1776 Massachusetts Avenue, N.W., Washington, D.C. 20036. The association is engaged in a continuing series of studies on disability research on behalf of the National Science Foundation. For reports on their projects and for papers they have compiled from their many workshops on the subject, contact Dr. Martha Ross Redden at AAAS.

4. Forty thousand dollars seems like a lot of money to spend on rehabilitation of a single individual. Howard Rusk does not think it is. He told the Subcommittee on Select Education in 1978: "This is looking at the problem from the cold economic angle, leaving the most important factor out of the consideration, and that is the human being, his potential, his right to live the best life he can with what he has left. . . . If we do not give them the opportunity to live productive lives, if this is possible, they will grow up to say, 'You have kept us alive, for what?' "

5. Kao's work was reported by Colen in the November 7, 1978, Washington *Post*, A3.
6. For information on the NYU electronic wheelchair, write to the Institute of Rehabilitation Medicine, 400 E. 34th Street, New York, New York 10016.
7. On limb regeneration, see "Advances in Limb Regeneration Reported," Washington *Star*, August 21, 1978, A12.
8. Persons interested in mental retardation "cures" may write to the National Association for Retarded Citizens, 2709 Avenue E East, Arlington, Texas 76011.
9. Klein's article appeared in the Washington *Post*, August 29, 1978, on the op-ed page. For an extended discussion of the entire issue of ethics in biology and other life sciences, I recommend two sources in particular. One is *Science* magazine, which has carried stories on bioethics for several years. The other is *Hastings Center Report*. For a readable consideration of some of the broader issues, see Vance Packard's *The People Shapers* (1977). George F. Will discussed the ethics of sterilization of retarded persons in the Washington *Post*, December 3, 1978, C7.
10. The U.S. Office of Education, under the guidance of Dr. Edwin W. Martin, has attempted for several years to convince the commercial networks to caption television programs. Eventually, Martin was forced to give up on open captions and press for closed captions. Even here, the networks gave him a very hard time. Because he has had to fight so hard, Martin has become an expert on the question. Write to him at USOE, Donohue Building, Washington, D.C. 20202.

Chapter 3. The Barriers Come Tumbling Down

1. The George F. Will quote is from a column of his in the Washington *Post*, May 5, 1977.
2. Larry Wiseman reported on the Shriners' performance at RFK Stadium in an article entitled, "Toward Respect, Not Charity, for the Disabled," in the Washington *Post*, August 30, 1977, on the op-ed page.

3. The Burger quote is from his decision on *Griggs,* 401 U.S. 424 (1971).

4. For samples of the section 504 controversy coverage in the press, see: Crosby's Washington *Star* story, "Mass Transit's Emotional Blockbuster," September 14, 1978, A1, C8. Crosby quotes from testimony on the Department of Transportation's section 504 regulation; *U.S. News & World Report,* "What's Being Done for 35 Million Handicapped," August 29, 1977, 58; Stanfield (1978); Clark (1978); and two New York *Times* articles by Steven V. Roberts (1978 a, b).

5. For information on the Pennhurst case, contact Thomas Gilhool, Counsel, Public Interest Law Center of Philadelphia, 1315 Walnut Street, Philadelphia, Pennsylvania 19107. Gilhool represented the plaintiffs in the case. He was also the counsel for the plaintiffs in the *Pennsylvania Association for Retarded Citizens (P.A.R.C.) v. Pennsylvania* case that led to P.L. 94–142.

6. The Transbus controversy attracted considerable press attention. The public hearing records from the Transportation Department's 1978 regional hearings are available for public inspection. In addition to Roberts's and Crosby's stories, see two *Congressional Quarterly* stories by Arieff (1978 a, b); a Philadelphia *Inquirer* story by Representative Robert Edgar (D-PA) (1978); and *Business Week,* "Transbus Delay Hurts the Bus Makers," June 19, 1978, 27–28.

7. Neal Pierce's column in the Washington *Post,* "The Great Wheelchair Flap," appeared on the op-ed page, December 28, 1978. My response, "Civil Rights for the Disabled," is on the op-ed page of the *Post,* January 9, 1979. See also "Now, Wheelchair Rights," *Newsweek,* January 15, 1979, 37.

Chapter 4. Reaching for Potential

1. A good summary of the provisions of P.L. 94–142 may be found in Barbacovi & Clelland (1978). A readable and brief article by Zettel (1979) is also helpful. For further information about the law, contact the Council for Exceptional Children, 1920 Association Drive, Reston, Virginia 22091.

2. A very useful discussion of vocational education for disabled children may be found in Razeghi & Halloran (1978). For a book-length treatment, see Halloran, Foley, Razeghi & Hull (1978) and Phelps & Lutz (1977). For information on Marc Gold's work, write to him at the Institute for Child Behavior and Development, 51 Gerty Drive, Champaign, Illinois 61820.

3. Porter's columns appeared in the Washington *Star* in September, 1976, and on different dates in other newspapers across the country. If you cannot locate copies, write to the American Coalition of Citizens with Disabilities, Washington, D.C. 20005.

4. On the governors' opposition to rehabilitation and barrier removal, see Barnes's December 21, 1978, Washington *Star* story on page A4. Barnes concludes: "But there was a bright side for the President as well. He met with a half-dozen governors for an hour yesterday [December 20] and they endorsed his plan for fighting inflation by cutting the budget. They just asked for consolidated federal programs and delays in federally mandated spending for such things as the removal of architectural barriers to the handicapped. That is the kind of talk Carter likes." The Washington *Post* ran a story by Edward Walsh and David Broder December 21, 1978, reporting on the same meeting Barnes covered. According to the *Post* story, National Governors Association Chairman Julian M. Carroll, governor of Kentucky, "said the governors' support is 'absolutely' contingent upon consolidation and other steps that would reduce administrative costs to the states. He cited, as an example of programs mandated by Congress that might be delayed, requirements to remove architectural barriers to the handicapped in public buildings, which he said would cost more than $50 million in Kentucky alone." James Hyatt, writing in the *Wall Street Journal*, September 7, 1978, covered the NGA Boston meeting and the adoption of Governor Brown's "real Truth in Spending Act" resolution. He quoted another governor as saying about the governors' opposition to federal mandates

for which federal support is less than 100% of the costs: "I'll give you an example of the worst sort—education for the handicapped. But who can say anything against it? . . . That program alone, if fully carried out, would wreck the state treasury."

5. Jack Anderson's *Post* column on the administration's opposition to rehabilitation appeared January 24, 1979, B13, and was entitled, "Carter's Deal to Gut Aid Program." He also appeared on "Good Morning America" on August 24 and November 6 to discuss rehabilitation funding.

Chapter 5. Dependence and Independence

1. Kennedy made these remarks before the NGA Boston meeting, August 26, 1978.
2. On social-security expenditures on disability, see in particular Berkowitz, Johnson, & Murphy (1976), Berkowitz et al. (1978), and Treitel (1977). The annual reports of the board of trustees of SSA are excellent also.
3. These proposals for reforming the SSDI system have been suggested by a number of observers. I found legislative proposals developed by HEW for 1979 and 1980 very helpful in attaching cost figures to some of the alternatives. See also Berkowitz et al. (1978) and testimony presented on S. 2505 on September 26, 1978, by representatives of disabled people. The latter is available from the office of Senator Daniel Patrick Moynihan (D-NY).
4. On health-care costs and disability, two good sources are Duchnok (1978) and Ferron (1977). Milius (1979) is also helpful.
5. For more information on how much a person would have to earn to purchase adequate medical care, see in particular Turem (1975).
6. Lynn Thompson's story appeared in the Los Angeles *Times* and *Herald Examiner*, March 8, 1978. See Knowles and Townsend.
7. The Regional Rehabilitation Research Institute on Attitudi-

nal, Legal and Leisure Barriers (1828 L Street, N.W., Washington, D.C. 20036) has an excellent series of simple brochures on attitudes toward disability. For an outstanding film about attitudes toward employment of disabled persons, contact the President's Committee on Employment of the Handicapped, asking for *A Different Approach*. The Architectural and Transportation Barriers Compliance Board has a short brochure, "About Barriers."

8. For more information about legal rights of disabled people, contact the Public Interest Law Center of Philadelphia, or the National Center on Law and the Handicapped, Suite 1900, American National Bank Building, South Bend, Indiana 46601.

References

"Advances in Limb Regeneration Reported." Washington *Star*, August 21, 1978, A12.

Arieff, I. "General Motors, Elderly and Handicapped Groups Accept Transbus Plan." *Congressionl Quarterly*, September 6, 1978, 2446–47 (a).

Arieff, I. "Senate Panels Back Carter on Need to Revise Highway, Mass Transit Programs." *Congressional Quarterly*, June 10, 1978, 1476–77 (b).

Barbacovi, D., & Clelland, R. *Public Law 94–142: Special Education in Transition.* Arlington, VA: American Association of School Administrators, 1978.

Barnes, F. "President Gave Mayors Forum for Complaints." Washington *Star*, December 21, 1978, A4.

Berkowitz, M., Horning, M., McConnell, S., & Worrall, J. *Rehabilitating Social Security Disability Insurance Beneficiaries: The Promise and the Performance.* New Brunswick, NJ: Rutgers University Bureau of Economic Research, 1978.

Berkowitz, M., Johnson, W., & Murphy, E. *Public Policy toward Disability.* New York: Praeger, 1976.

Berkowitz, M., & Rubin, J. *The Costs of Disability: Estimates of Program Expenditures for Disability, 1967–1975.* New Brunswick, NJ: Bureau of Economic Research, 1977.

Boothroyd, A. "Technology and Deafness." *Volta Review*, January, 1975, 27–33.

Bowe, F. "Civil Rights of the Disabled." Washington *Post,* January 9, 1979, op-ed.

Bowe, F. "49 Days." *Equal Opportunity Forum,* July, 1977, 4–5.

Bowe, F. *Handicapping America.* New York: Harper & Row, 1978.

Bowe, F. "Looking beyond the Disabilities." *Worklife,* May, 1977, 13–15.

Bowe, F. "Who Are the Handicapped?" *Journal of Current Social Issues,* Spring, 1979, 4–7.

Bowe, F., Jacobi, J., & Wiseman, L. *Coalition Building.* Washington, D.C.: American Coalition of Citizens with Disabilities, Inc., 1978.

Bowe, F., & Williams, J. *Planning Effective Advocacy Programs.* Washington, D.C.: American Coalition of Citizens with Disabilities, Inc., 1979.

Burdette, M., & Frohlich, P. *The Effect of Disability in Unit Income: 1972 Survey of Disabled and Nondisabled Adults.* Report No. 9. Washington, D.C.: Social Security Administration, 1977.

Burdette, M., Frohlich, P., & Posner, I. *Work Disability in the United States: A Chartbook.* Washington, D.C.: U.S. Government Printing Office, 1977.

Califano, J. "The Aging of America." Remarks before the Academy of Political and Social Science, Philadelphia, Pennsylvania, April 8, 1978.

Califano, J. "Remarks before the Economic Club of Chicago." Mimeo. Washington, D.C.: U.S. Department of Health, Education, and Welfare, 1978.

Caplan, A., & Ordahl, C. "Irreversible Gene Repression Model for Control of Development." *Science,* July 14, 1978, 120–30.

Clark, T. "Access for the Handicapped: A Test of Carter's War on Inflation." *National Journal,* October 21, 1978, 1672–75.

Cohen, W. "Social Security: Focusing on the Facts." *AFL-CIO American Federationist,* April, 1978, 6-10.

Colen, B. "Success in Spinal Cord Repair Reported by GU Medical Team." Washington *Post,* November 7, 1978, A3.

Crosby, T. "Mass Transit's Emotional Blockbuster." Washington *Star,* September 14, 1978, A1, C8.

David, G. "Get Rich Quick: Train the Disabled." Philadelphia *Sunday Bulletin*, December 4, 1977, 1, 4.

Duchnok, S. *Health Care Coverage and Medical Care Utilization.* Report No. 11, August, 1978. Washington, D.C.: Social Security Administration, 1978.

Dudek, R. (ed) *Human Rehabilitation Techniques.* Final Report, vol. 1, part A. Lubbock, TX: Texas Tech University, 1978.

Edgar, R. "The Bill for the Handicapped Comes Too High." Philadelphia *Inquirer*, July 9, 1978, op-ed.

Elmes, D. (ed) *National Health Care Policies for the Handicapped: An Analysis of Selected Problem Areas Identified at the White House Conference on Handicapped Individuals.* Mimeo. Washington, D.C.: The White House, 1978.

Ferron, D. *Medical Care Charges for the Disabled and Nondisabled.* Report No. 7, October, 1977. Washington, D.C.: Social Security Administration, 1977.

Franklin, P. "Impact of Disability on the Family Structure." *Social Security Bulletin*, May, 1977, 3–18.

Franklin, P. "Impact of Substantial Gainful Activity Level on Disabled Beneficiary Work Patterns." *Social Security Bulletin*, August, 1976, 21–30.

Freebairn, T. *Telecommunications and Deafness: The State of the Art.* New York: Deafness Research & Training Center, 1976.

Freiberger, H., Sherrick, C., & Scadden, L. *Report on the Workshop on Sensory Deficits and Sensory Aids.* Mimeo, 1977.

Frohlich, P., & Schechter, E. *Assets and Disability.* Report No. 8, November, 1977. Washington, D.C.: Social Security Administration, 1977.

Halloran, W., Foley, T., Razeghi, J., & Hull, M. *Vocational Education for the Handicapped: Resource Guide to the Regulations.* Austin, TX: Texas Regional Resource Center (201 E. Eleventh Street, Austin, TX 78701), 1978.

Hooker, M., & Krute, A. "Disabled Worker Beneficiaries under OASDI: Comparison with Severely Disabled PA Recipients." *Social Security Bulletin*, August, 1977, 15–22.

Hudson, R. "Political and Budgetary Consequences of an Aging Population." *National Journal*, October 21, 1978, 1699–1705.

Hyatt, J. "Congress Mandates Laws but States Pay for Them." *Wall Street Journal*, September 7, 1978.

Kerr, C., & Rosow, J. (ed) *Work in America: The Decade Ahead.* New York: Van Nostrand Reinhold, 1978.

Klein, R. "The New Life-or-Death Choices." Washington *Post*, August 29, 1978, op-ed.

Knowles, R. "A Woman's Suicide: 'Thanks for Being the Straw that Broke the Camel's Back.' " Los Angeles *Herald Examiner*, March 8, 1978.

Krute, A., & Burdette, E. *Chronic Disease, Injury, and Work Disability.* Report No. 10, April, 1978. Washington, D.C.: Social Security Administration, 1978.

McCormack, P. "Access for the Handicapped: A 'Now' Concern." Boston *Herald American*, September 11, 1977.

Meyers, R. *Like Other People.* New York: McGraw-Hill, 1978.

Milius, P. "Social Security: Some Good News." Washington *Post*, February 6, 1979, Al.

Moseley, R. "Gaps in Medicare Trap the Elderly." Chicago *Tribune*, September 28, 1978, 1, 6.

Nicholson, R. "Human Factors and the Handicapped." *Human Factors*, 1978, 20(3), 259–72.

Orin, D. "Scandal School Shut after Losing Funding." New York *Post*, December 7, 1977, 10.

Packard, V. *The People Shapers.* Boston: Little, Brown, 1977.

Pierce, N. "The Great Wheelchair Flap." Washington *Post*, December 28, 1978, op-ed.

Phelps, A. & Lutz, R. *Career Exploration and Preparation for the special Needs Learner.* Rockleigh. NJ: Allyn & Bacon, 1977.

Pines, M. "Modern Bioengineers Reinvent Human Anatomy with Spare Parts." *Smithsonian*, vol. 9, no. 8, August, 1978, 50–56.

Posner, *Functional Capacity Limitations and Disability, 1972.* Report No. 2, March, 1977. Washington, D.C.: Social Security Administration, 1977.

Razeghi, J., & Halloran, W. "A New Picture of Vocational Education for the Employment of the Handicapped." *School Shop*, April, 1978, 50–43.

Roberts, S. "The Handicapped are Emerging as a Vocal Political Action Group." *New York Times,* June 19, 1978, A16–17 (a).

Roberts, S. "Putting a Price Tag on Equality." *New York Times,* June 25, 1978 (b).

Robertson, A. *The Financial Status of Social Security after the Social Security Amendments of 1977.* Washington, D.C.: Social Security Administration, 1978.

Samuelson, R. "Busting the U.S. Budget—The Costs of an Aging America." *National Journal,* February 18, 1978, 256–60.

Schechter, E. *Employment and Work Adjustment of the Disabled.* Washington, D.C.: Social Security Administration, 1977.

Stanfield, R. "Bringing the World to the Disabled—The Feds Start to Get Tough." *National Journal,* February 18, 1978, 272–76.

Townsend, D. "Suicide Spurs Disabled to Ask End to Funds Cutoff." Los Angeles *Times,* March 8, 1978.

"Transit and the Handicapped." Washington *Star* editorial, September 18, 1978.

Treitel, R. *Rehabilitation of Disabled Adults, 1972.* Report No. 3, May, 1977. Washington, D.C.: Social Security Administration, 1977.

Turem, J. (ed) *Report of the Comprehensive Service Needs Study.* Washington, D.C.: The Urban Institute, 1975.

Walsh, E., & Broder, D. "Mayors, Governors See Carter; Press Cases on '80 Budget." Washington *Post,* December 21, 1978, A2.

"When Disability Pay Starts to Hurt." Washington *Post,* January 12, 1978, A26.

Will, G. "Sterilization and the Retarded." Washington *Post,* December 3, 1978, C7.

Will, G. "Sympathetic Justice." Washington *Post,* May 5, 1977.

Witt, E. "Disability Aid Serious Drain on Economy." Washington *Post,* December 19, 1977.

Zettel, J. "Disabled Children and the Path to Equal Educational Opportunity." *Equa! Opportunity Forum,* February, 1979, 6–7, 23.

Index